Healing

Finding Satisfaction in a Healthcare Career

MARK TOPAZIAN

Purpose

ĩvp
Academic
An imprint of InterVarsity Press
Downers Grove, Illinois

InterVarsity Press
P.O. Box 1400 | Downers Grove, IL 60515-1426
ivpress.com | email@ivpress.com

InterVarsity Press® is the publishing division of InterVarsity Christian Fellowship/USA®. For more information, visit intervarsity.org.

All Scripture quotations, unless otherwise indicated, are taken from The Holy Bible, New International Version®, NIV®. Copyright © 1973, 1978, 1984, 2011 by Biblica, Inc.™ Used by permission of Zondervan. All rights reserved worldwide. www.zondervan.com. The "NIV" and "New International Version" are trademarks registered in the United States Patent and Trademark Office by Biblica, Inc.™

While any stories in this book are true, some names and identifying information have been changed to protect the privacy of individuals.

The publisher cannot verify the accuracy or functionality of website URLs used in this book beyond the date of publication.

Cover design: Faceout Studio, Jeff Miller
Interior design: Jeanna Wiggins
Images: Getty Images: © oxygen / Moment; © bortonia / DigitalVision Vectors

ISBN 978-1-5140-1238-3 (print) | ISBN 978-1-5140-1239-0 (digital)

Printed in the United States of America ♾

Library of Congress Cataloging-in-Publication Data
A catalog record for this book is available from the Library of Congress.

32 31 30 29 28 27 26 25 | 12 11 10 9 8 7 6 5 4 3 2 1

"I first met Mark Topazian when we shared a room in a Muslim family's home after the fall of the Albanian dictatorship that had made God illegal for a generation. He has worked most of his career as a Mayo Clinic physician and has more recently served in healthcare ministry in Ethiopia. I bring this up to focus on his authenticity and authority to speak for both science and faith. He has done so beautifully in this biblically grounded, scientifically accurate work that guides us and compels us to seek the wonderful wholeness that God has planned for us and those we serve."

Al Weir, author of *When Your Doctor Has Bad News* and former president of the Christian Medical and Dental Associations

"Mark Topazian's book does accomplish its purpose. His honest and forthright accounts of patient encounters and a search for spiritual meaning in our work did indeed fan the flames of my own passion to practice nursing as ministry. There are reflection and application exercises at the end of each chapter to personalize learning. Dr. Topazian makes us feel it is okay to struggle, to doubt, to embrace our calling, and to use our faith as a resource to combat fatigue and burnout. This book is a breath of fresh air for all those called to ministry in healthcare."

Kristen L. Mauk, professor and associate dean of graduate studies and research at Colorado Christian University and coeditor of *Nursing as Ministry*

"Globally, training in the healthcare disciplines typically excludes the acknowledgment of God as Creator, source of all wisdom, and the ultimate healer. In *Healing Purpose*, Mark Topazian uses his personal experience, numerous references, and biblical truth to fill this gap in our understanding and practice of medical science. He provides a sound context for those who desire to practice their noble professions to their full potential in promoting health and caring for the sick, in the way God intended."

Keith Michael, CEO of Healthcare Christian Fellowship International

"Those of us who work in healthcare have an incredible opportunity to follow in the footsteps of Jesus when we bring hope and healing to our patients, but it's not always easy to do so when we are confronted with overwhelming suffering and crushed under heavy workloads. This book examines the many challenges that faithful practitioners face and provides practical guidance on how to overcome them."

Matthew Loftus, author and family physician at PCEA Chogoria Hospital in Kenya

"Dr. Mark Topazian weaves together powerful clinical stories, biblical accounts, and evidence-based research to insightfully describe the need we all have to receive holistic care. He gives us concise and accessible ways to integrate Christian faith into our daily work in healthcare. From practicing repentance and lament to praying with patients, Dr. Topazian offers practical next steps for those seeking to discover deeper meaning and purpose in their work. I am excited to share this book with healthcare students, faculty, and professionals!"

Renee Nicholas, national director of InterVarsity Graduate Healthcare Ministries

"*Healing Purpose* provides much-needed insight and awareness regarding the importance of addressing our patients and ourselves as whole beings—mind, body, and spirit. Too often, we feel unprepared to assess and address the spiritual needs of others. We close off these parts of ourselves as burnout and compassion fatigue take hold. This book fills in the gaps and provides a primer for balanced, whole-person care. It sees each of us for all that we are."

Christy Secor, director and spiritual formation and prayer specialist for the Nurses Christian Fellowship

"God has graciously gifted me with a longtime friendship and fellowship with Dr. Mark Topazian. In these pages, Mark conveys a biblical understanding of God's purpose for healing the sick, garnered from decades of patient care as a Christ-follower in academic medicine. Medicine has been a powerful tool in his life as a gastroenterologist to introduce patients to a healing God. Mark reminds us that all healing is the result of God's common grace, and we, as healthcare professionals, are ministers of that common grace. We have daily opportunities to point patients and their families to the author and sustainer of shalom in our own lives and the lives of those entrusted to our care. Mark also reminds us that restoring whole health to patients (i.e., body, soul, and spirit) brings some of the greatest joy to a healthcare professional's life. Because this is true, we *must* do a better job equipping the next generation of Christian healthcare professionals to address this holistic care. *Healing Purpose* is a book that I would urge every Christian medical or dental trainee (student, resident, or fellow) in the US or around the globe to read before they graduate or start their practice."

Mike Chupp, CEO of the Christian Medical and Dental Associations

In memory of my dad,
David S. Topazian, DDS,

who modeled for me a purposeful
and satisfying healthcare career.

Contents

Acknowledgments

THIS BOOK HAS MANY SOURCES. Throughout my medical career I've learned from colleagues, mentors, and patients who have shown me how to find satisfaction in healthcare practice. This book belongs to them.

I'm grateful to my wife, Janet, my kindred spirit and partner in life, who helped launch and sustain this project, and to our daughters, Hillary, Rachel, and Elise. Their encouragement made this book possible. I also thank the medical students, residents, nurses, and therapists from various faith traditions who explored many of this book's topics with me during summertime Bible studies in Rochester, Minnesota. Their questions and insights about medicine and spirituality shaped my approach to this book.

My friend Dr. Joe Sprinkle, an Old Testament professor, has given me counsel and theological direction starting with the first version of this material. Dr. Dennis Palmer and Dr. Greg Kline also offered helpful guidance at early stages. Professor Mark Talbot kindly read portions of my draft manuscript, shared his insights with me, and gave me helpful advice. Dr. Barney Davis suggested the title for chapter ten, and Drs. Susan Kok, Eric McLaughlin, Rachel Nunn, Emily Potter, Hillary Topazian, and Al Weir prompted important revisions to the manuscript. IHS Global, which stewards the Saline Process Witness Training program, graciously gave me permission to adapt portions of the Saline Process curriculum in this book. You can learn more about Saline Process at https://ihsglobal.org/salineprocess.

I'm indebted to Colton Bernasol and Rebecca Carhart, my editors at InterVarsity Press, for their expert guidance. Thank you both!

Introduction

WHEN I STARTED IN HEALTHCARE, nothing made me happier than making sick people better. Establishing a diagnosis, applying an effective treatment, and seeing the patient improve was a rewarding cycle that I repeated over and over again. The successful practice of modern medicine is addictive; we health workers accomplish good things for our patients while enjoying their gratitude and reveling in our own skills.[1] A friend of mine gave up rock climbing after becoming a surgeon. He no longer felt the urge to climb because he got the same rush as a surgeon that he'd experienced on the cliffs.

To this day I typically leave work happy because I've helped my patients. But I've discovered that there is danger in relying on clinical success for my professional satisfaction. For one thing, success becomes routine. The hundredth time we cure pneumonia or repair a hernia or deliver a baby it's not as thrilling as it was the first time. In many situations, good outcomes become an expectation, not a source of gratification. And when there is too much work, success can become an exhausting demand. What's more, treatment success is an unstable basis for satisfaction in healthcare because it can depend on clinical circumstances beyond our control. When we come to know ourselves primarily as successful clinicians—not as sons or daughters, partners, friends, children of God—our self-identity increasingly rests on an unstable foundation. It's like a house built on sand. We may struggle with anxiety or anger when good patient outcomes elude us, and we may deal poorly with some patients, to our own detriment. A patient I once referred for surgery was worse off after his operation, and the surgeon was uninterested in following up with him. I was left managing his condition. One day the patient told me that, as they passed each other in the hallways of our facility, the surgeon had glanced at him and then looked away. For my colleague the patient was an unpleasant reminder of his own limitations, but my patient felt abandoned. A lawsuit followed.

I found a different pathway to satisfaction in healthcare early in my practice as a gastroenterologist. A patient of mine was hospitalized with pancreatitis caused by an endoscopic procedure I'd performed. I had informed her of the possibility beforehand, but she was nevertheless sick thanks to me. I felt responsible for her illness and dreaded visiting her hospital room each morning. I would steel myself, walk in, greet her, and move her bedside tray so that I could examine her. I would then force myself to sit down and linger at her bedside. I learned about her work and family. I discovered her generosity of spirit. I took care of her. Over ten days she gradually got better. To my surprise I found that not only was our relationship intact following this episode, but it was stronger than before. She sent me a gift at Christmas. Of all the patients I treated that year, she is the one I most remember, the one who ultimately brought me the most satisfaction.

Standing by a patient and their family—even when things don't go well, or treatment options are inadequate, or they are difficult people—is exhausting for some healthcare professionals, but it has become a source of satisfaction for me. It requires a personal investment that doesn't always seem to pay off, at least not immediately. But the gratification that comes from serving others in challenging times is different from the fun of good outcomes. It develops slowly but lasts longer. It affirms not only my technical skill but also my humanity. During these times, my patients benefit when I treat them not just as bodies but as the tight-knit combination of body, soul, and spirit that they are. Treating them this way lifts me up too, because satisfaction is more

Satisfaction is more than happiness: it is the contentment, meaning, and fulfillment that come from engaging all of who I am in pursuit of something good.

than happiness; it is the contentment, meaning, and fulfillment that come from engaging all of who I am in pursuit of something good.

Standing by our patients is but one of many ways of finding fulfillment through the spiritual dimension of healthcare. Now, the very idea that medicine and spirituality mix may surprise you. Although most people believe in the existence of a spiritual reality, we often have a hard time linking meaning and matter, faith and science, our inner sense of personal connection to the divine and our outward roles in society. While working in healthcare, I've often experienced this tension. I tend toward a dual existence: spiritually minded at home and at church, scientifically minded at work.

My own journey toward recognizing spiritual realities in the hospital began when I was a third-year medical student. I had heard that the chief resident running a service I was assigned to was, like me, a Christian, and I figured that he would know some of the secrets of integrating faith and practice. I asked him whether he could tell me how to be a Christian in healthcare. "Let's meet a half hour before rounds tomorrow and pray through our team's patient list together," he said. His response disappointed me. It seemed too simple. But I could hardly turn down his invitation! We met the next morning in a small room on the medical ward. As we prayed for the patients on our list, I experienced the presence of God with us—a presence I had sometimes felt when praying at home or in church but never before in the hospital. It dawned on me that I had been leaving God at the door of the hospital when I walked through it each morning wearing my white coat. As we rounded that morning, I saw our patients differently. They were more than their problem lists. They were, like me, God's good and everlasting creation.

Since then, on my best days, I'm aware that God is in the hospital. I've come to understand that he is near to my patients and active in my clinic, and that my patients and I both benefit when I recognize his presence. The joy that comes from experiencing God at work is available to me on good days, bad days, and routine days. It is usually triggered by clinical events and patient encounters, but it is independent of clinical outcomes. It is satisfying because it brings meaning to what I do. It is sustaining because it connects me in real time to God's purpose, power, and love.

There are obstacles to experiencing the spiritual dimension of our work. Healthcare can be so busy that sometimes there simply seems to be no space in our workflow for God. And if you're like me, you've wondered whether your worldview has any standing in the halls of a hospital, where biomedical evidence is the basis for our work and there is typically no consensus about faith. Maybe you believe that eternal souls are what really matter in the long run but think that at work we are only treating mortal bodies. For some of us, our spiritual sensitivity has atrophied, and we're less able to perceive the significance of our work—just as people who've lost their sense of smell have trouble tasting food. Practically speaking, many of us find it easy to converse with our patients about medical topics, but we feel uncomfortable asking about their emotions and their spirituality. For all of these reasons it's easy to practice the healing arts while only dimly aware of the immaterial dimensions of our work. Yet in doing so we miss out on much of the satisfaction our work can bring us.

For me, recognizing God's presence is not about extended periods of meditation or prayer during my workday. There isn't time for those. Snatches of prayer, Scripture, and song do come to my mind at work, and I think it's possible to prepare ourselves ahead of time to experience those when we need them most. But often, recognizing the spiritual dimensions of clinical scenarios is what connects me to God. He is not a distraction from our work or ancillary to our work. He is present in our work. Discovering him in the middle of our workflow can bring us joy.

What does that look like? Last week I was asked to see a boy who could no longer attend school because of an undiagnosed illness. He had already been evaluated by multiple specialists, and I was doubtful that I could help.

> God is not a distraction from our work or ancillary to our work. He is present in our work.

I thought I had forestalled the consult, but there he was: the last patient on my Monday afternoon clinic list. His father carried him into my exam room. After introductions I began taking his medical history. When I got to the social history, I asked about his school and his family. Then I asked his father,

"Is faith a part of your family life?" I was seeing them in a secular healthcare setting where faith is rarely talked about, but I know that it's best medical practice to ask this. The father looked at me, surprised. None of the preceding consultants had asked him this question. "We're Muslim," he said. "Has your faith community supported you as you've gone through all this?" I asked. "Oh, they've been helpful," he said. "That's good," I responded, and then I moved on to questions about the family medical history.

By the time I was examining the boy, the annoyance I had felt was gone and compassion was stirring in my heart. As things wrapped up, I put my arm around the boy's shoulder and said to him and his father, "You've seen a lot of doctors and don't have answers yet. I don't know if I will find an answer either, but I know our Creator has the answers." For the first time in our meeting, the father smiled and nodded.

I will see the boy and his father next week in follow-up. I'm still waiting for test results, and I don't know whether I will make a diagnosis or whether spirituality will surface again when we meet. But I've already found satisfaction in caring for this boy.

The brief spiritual history that I took reminded me that God was present in my exam room and had a purpose for our encounter that I've yet to discover. I relaxed as I aligned with God: this boy's outcome is in his hands, not mine, and my responsibility is to play my part with excellence. I began to wonder what intention our loving God has for this boy and his father. I remembered that I can choose to be salt and light in unsavory and dim situations. I regained, in my clinic, the perspective and purpose of a child of God.

We rightly aim to find satisfaction in our work (Eccles 2:24; 3:12-13; Is 55:1-2; Jn 10:10). But some of us are running on empty, and our own sense of meaning and purpose has been slipping away. Maybe, like me, you've gone through seasons when work is emotionally draining or boring, or seems unrewarding apart from your paycheck. Imagine, then, absorbing a patient's suffering at close range and experiencing God's comfort in return instead of caregiving fatigue. Or, when work is routine, discovering variety and opportunity in the spirits of the people around you. Or, when things are not going your way, feeling peace instead of frustration or anger. Perceiving God while at work and knowing him through our work renews our purpose and leads to professional fulfillment in all of these situations.

The goal of this book is to refresh your calling to healthcare and rekindle your joy in your work.[2] Equitable working conditions, acceptable working hours, and a supportive and healthy workplace culture all help to sustain us through our healthcare careers—but these alone will not bring us satisfaction. The premise of this book is that, to a surprising extent, healthcare careers are most fulfilling when we recognize and embrace the spiritual aspect of our profession. If you're suffering from compassion fatigue, this book will help you recover a healthy perspective on your work—and decide what needs to change. If you're content professionally, this book will open your eyes to the deeper purpose of your day-to-day routine and to new ways to thrive. If you're a student or trainee learning a healthcare profession, this book offers a foundation for a satisfying career.

Spirituality has a place in healthcare because the scientific and spiritual accounts of personhood, sickness, and healing are actually one unified story of God's creative and redemptive work in human lives. Understanding this unified narrative reframes our understanding of our work, changes how we interact with our patients, and gives us resources to cope with the demands healthcare places on us. To explore this story and its importance for our careers, we're going to look at biblical concepts and practical methods that are highly relevant to our work. We'll find that the Bible has a lot to say about health, sickness, and healing, and that biomedical science and ancient scriptural texts are compatible. However, the goal of this exploration is not only to study ideas but to show how our faith matters at work and equips us to excel at and enjoy our jobs. Understanding how your faith syncs with your work will give you opportunities to find greater fulfillment in healthcare.

As a Christian, I see these topics through a biblical lens. If you too are a Christian, this book will challenge you to approach your work in new ways. If you are curious about Christianity, give this book a try! It offers a different perspective on why you do what you do, rooted in texts people have looked to for guidance for millennia. In either case, this book will help you clarify and expand the meaning and purpose of your work in healthcare.

This book has four sections. In the first section, we'll look at a biblical understanding of anatomy: not our tissues and organ systems, but the way body, soul, and spirit, fused together and made in God's image, define who we and our patients are. The significance of our work comes fully into view when we appreciate the full dimensionality of human beings. In the second section, we'll consider how biblical perspectives on health, sickness, and healing shape our purpose and shift our approach to our work. We'll also discover how the subconscious fear of death can steal our professional satisfaction, and what we can do about it.

In the third section, we'll consider the impact that patients' suffering and taxing clinical scenarios have on our well-being. The accumulated burden we end up carrying is a major source of compassion fatigue, and the work of bearing it leads some of us to leave patient care. The Bible depicts healthy ways of dealing with the weight of caregiving—responses that can mitigate our compassion fatigue, increase our professional satisfaction, and even revitalize our own spiritual lives. In the fourth and final section, we'll explore the connections between the Christian gospel, healing, and faith. We'll see that healthcare work is properly understood as gospel work and that God is using us every day in our healthcare contexts. Aligning ourselves with that reality renews our healing purpose.

Of course, ideas alone won't transform your work life. Just as new scientific discoveries only change healthcare practice once they're applied in clinical settings, propositions about spirituality and healthcare only affect us when we apply them to our daily experience. Each chapter concludes with reflection questions that groups can use and exercises that aim to enhance the satisfaction we get from our work. Pick the exercise at the end of each chapter that seems most relevant to you and practice it before moving on. These exercises require effort, but they are key to experiencing the benefits this book talks about.

God has given you your heart, knowledge, skills, and personality. He is already using you where he has placed you. I hope that this book will fan into flame your calling to healthcare, open your eyes to God's active presence in your workplace, and bring you joy!

PART 1

Anatomy

1

Being Human

DURING A RECENT DAY IN CLINIC, I was seeing a young woman to provide a second opinion about her medical situation.[1] I met her in a consultation room after reviewing a stack of her records. As she told me her medical history, I got the impression she was a bit witless: her narrative was punctuated by high-pitched giggles, and she had a hard time distinguishing her responses to the various treatments she had received. I looked again through the records she had brought, trying to distill a more complete understanding of her course. I asked some questions repeatedly: Had she felt better after surgery or not? Had a particular medication seemed helpful to her? She had a hard time telling. I found the interview frustrating.

I asked whether she worked. She told me that she was employed at a development project targeting at-risk youth. I asked her to tell me more. The giggles disappeared from her speech as her passion for children and her pride in her work spilled out in my exam room. It became clear that she was committed to making the world a better place. I was impressed by what she was accomplishing in spite of her medical situation. I realized that she was brave, and I told her so. My first impression of her was wrong. I had missed the person hidden behind the medical facts.

I saw her again after her test results were back, and we decided on a treatment plan. I asked her whether she wanted to return to the care of the physician who had been treating her. She paused, ambivalent. "I respect his knowledge and skills, but he treats me like I'm an idiot," she said.

We healthcare professionals deal with human beings. As we see more and more of them, they can become for us mainly problems to solve or objects to fix: the headache in the next examining bay or the gallbladder in room 23. I've worked in more than twenty hospitals and many clinics in a variety of healthcare contexts, both secular and faith based, on two continents, and I know that patients can easily become commodities in all sorts of practice settings. I've visited clinics where the caregivers only briefly made eye contact with their clients, instead focusing their attention on particular body parts, test reports, prescription writing, and order entry as they made their way through lengthy lists of patients. Similarly, nurses working understaffed shifts tell me the pace of their work leaves no time for conversations with their patients. As our patients become commodities, we can lose sight of their humanity and can even come to resent them—particularly the ones who seem to be wasting our time, and especially when we're fatigued and overworked. A colleague of mine, near the end of a hectic month in his second year of residency, was able to catch a few hours of sleep. He dreamed he was assessing a new patient in the emergency department. In his dream he reached for the wall-mounted ophthalmoscope above the patient's gurney, only to find it was a gun.

Few of us went into healthcare expecting it would be like this. But there are many reasons it can turn out this way—reasons found within ourselves, our patients, our culture, and the structure of the systems we work in. Underlying all of these reasons are basic assumptions about the nature of human beings. The path to a satisfying healthcare career requires livable work schedules, acceptable working conditions, help with moral injury and other stresses when needed, and adequate time for the rest of our lives—but these alone don't bring us fulfillment at work. If our patients are commodities, then we are too, and healthcare practice becomes primarily an economic activity, an exchange of goods and services, a business in which efficiency and throughput are not only important but paramount.

> As our patients become commodities, we can lose sight of their humanity and can even come to resent them.

Having a beneficial purpose in life is associated, on average, with a longer and happier life.[2] To appreciate what our purpose is and how it sustains and benefits us, we need to ask why sick people are worth our time and effort. People are smarter than other living beings but cheetahs are faster, elephants are stronger, and undersea sponges and corals live much longer. In all these ways and more, species are different from each other. What, if anything, makes humans stand out from the rest of creation? And how does this influence our understanding of our purpose, our approach to our work, and the satisfaction we derive from caring for our patients?

GOD'S IMAGE

The story of our origins told in Genesis gives us insight into the essence of being human. In the biblical account, God speaks the animals into existence and tells them to teem, to "be fruitful and increase in number" (Gen 1:22). Then he creates humans:

> God said, "Let us make mankind in our image, in our likeness, so that they may rule over the fish in the sea and the birds in the sky, over the livestock and all the wild animals, and over all the creatures that move along the ground."
>
> So God created mankind in his own image,
> in the image of God he created them;
> male and female he created them.
>
> God blessed them and said to them, "Be fruitful and increase in number; fill the earth and subdue it. Rule over the fish in the sea and the birds in the sky and over every living creature that moves on the ground." (Gen 1:26-28)

According to this account, the first humans, like other living beings, were given a creaturely mandate to fill the earth, to have offspring, and create a society.[3] Biologist E. O. Wilson uses the term *sociobiology* to describe this persistent driver of both human and animal social behavior. But humans were also made "in the image of God," so that we can fulfill an additional mandate to "rule over" (or steward) creation. God's image grounds our identity and enables us to carry out this mandate.[4]

What does it mean to be made in God's image? Since God is spirit, it is probably not a reference to our physical form—but, as biological beings, we embody qualities of God that determine our nature and inform our place and role in the world.[5] The Bible nowhere concisely explains the concept of the image of God, but the text of Genesis gives us important clues. God's likeness, a unique feature of humans among all the created beings, is at the core of who we are and what we do. It imparts attributes, potential, and purpose to us, including the following.

Work. We were made in God's image so that we can rule over creation, meaning we're made to take responsibility for our world. Surprisingly, it's our work—not our religiosity—that is most directly linked to the image of God concept in Genesis 1. Our innate drive to accomplish tasks, pursue goals, and make progress is evidence of the image in which we were made. God performed the work of creation for six days and then gave humans a unique mandate to do the work of caring for what he had created. The animals weren't instructed to work. Our stewardship mandate was given to us just before God rested on the seventh day, as though he were passing the baton of creation care to Adam and Eve. We are designed to work, and work is an intrinsically good human activity, appointed before brokenness entered the human experience.

Our model for work is God himself. In Genesis 1 he uses his power to create a complex, harmonious, and sustainable world, full of abundance and potential, in which many different living things thrive. To rule over creation doesn't mean to prioritize our self-interest at the expense of the world around us. We are royal representatives tasked with tending creation with ingenuity and skill so that all of it will flourish. Tim Keller writes, "We are called to stand in for God here in the world, exercising stewardship over the rest of creation in his place as his vice-regents. We share in doing the things that God has done in creation—bringing order out of chaos, creatively building a civilization out of the material of physical and human nature, caring for all that God has made."[6] The image of God we bear enables us to work this way.

Healthcare work is Genesis 1 work. We restore God's creation by tending to human health. What's more, the image of God embedded in us finds expression as we practice our vocation. We can describe God's image in us as an angled mirror that reflects the love and care of God into the world.[7] When we use the power God has given us for the flourishing of others, we're reflecting the image of God into his creation.[8] In doing so we affirm our own identity, we fulfill the purpose God equipped us for, and we find significance in our work.

Creativity. God is the prime Creator. In the Genesis account we see him create a world of mind-boggling complexity, diversity, beauty, and balance. He delights in creation and excels at creation, and everything he creates is good.

Human creativity is an emblem of God's likeness. While there are examples of animals modifying found objects and then using them as basic tools, humans intentionally make new things as varied as furniture and pharmaceuticals, recipes and radio, symphonies and space telescopes. Adam uses his creativity to name the animals in Genesis 2. While his creative powers are on a completely different scale from God's (who made the animals) they set him in a middle ground between God and other living beings.

Creativity may be expressed in many ways—through music, art, writing, photography, crafts, humor, construction, gardening, landscaping, and cooking, to name a few examples. It finds expression in almost all human lives, especially when we are healthy. Creativity is one way for sick or disabled persons to express their humanity, and they may also connect with their identity when they enjoy the creative works of others. In healthcare, we use our creativity to find solutions to patient problems: we discover new treatments, adapt known methods to best suit the individual patient in front of us, and find new ways of encouraging the souls we care for. When our own lives are out of balance, practicing or experiencing human creativity can help us reclaim our own humanity.

Spirituality. We are spirits, and we can relate to other spirits, especially God. Because we're made in the image of God, our most basic relationship is upward with God himself.[9] In the first chapters of Genesis, Adam and Eve meet with God, walk with God in the garden, and have conversations with him. While animals also have spirits, the early chapters of Genesis do not show them interacting with God in the same way.[10] The human spirit is qualitatively different, as shown by our desire for meaning, our ability to intuit other spirits, and our capacity to communicate with God in prayer and worship.

We take for granted our ability to think, question, and communicate in propositional terms, and this fluency with meaning fills our days. Our lifelong search for personal meaning—for overarching matters of significance and purpose that go beyond ourselves—reveals our spiritual nature. In materialistic cultures, spirituality is often suppressed, and we can become spiritually dull: less able to know other people deeply, to experience God's presence, or to find significance in life. But even people who do not recognize spiritual reality, and believe we are no more than biological machines, experience the necessity of meaning. Spirituality explains why personal meaningfulness matters to us and why meaninglessness brings despair.[11] Data linking robust spirituality to improved health outcomes—which we'll explore later—validate the importance of the human spirit and its relevance to human well-being. In healthcare, recognizing the spiritual dimension of our work brings meaning to our day-to-day routine. That's why career fulfillment can come from perceiving God while we're at work and aligning ourselves with him.

Worth. The text of Genesis draws a parallel between the way Seth, Adam's son, carries his father's likeness and the way all of humanity carries God's image. It was not Adam and Eve alone who bore God's likeness; we all do. We have a family relationship with God (just as Seth did with Adam) because we are made in his image. We, in some sense, resemble God, and we can truly call him our father (Gen 5:1-3).[12]

The value this gives human beings is shown later on in Genesis, when God gives Noah and his children "everything that lives and moves about" for food, while at the same time stipulating that the killing of humans is punishable by death, "for in the image of God has God made mankind" (Gen 9:3, 6). The image of God is the basis for the respect we show other people, above and beyond the respect we show to animals.

The conviction that all persons are fundamentally equal springs from the belief that we all equally bear the image of God. This ethic does not come from science, which gives us normal distributions and the survival of the fittest—realities that are, by themselves, inadequate guides to our concept of human worth.[13] No matter our intelligence, beauty, charisma, athletic prowess, productivity, moral decency, or contribution to science or society, we're all equally made in God's image. We bear God's likeness from conception, and it remains with us, no matter how difficult or debilitated we become. Our belief in the intrinsic, equal worth of every human being is rooted in the Genesis account.

The equality of individuals is a core tenet of medical ethics, but research demonstrates that in practice we may treat patients unequally. Empirical studies show that we sometimes recommend lesser care to people who are different than we are due to their race, ethnicity, gender, culture, or socio-economic status, for instance when assessing and treating pain.[14] We don't mean to do this, but it may happen anyway, reflecting deep-seated elements of our outlook. Recognizing that all our patients bear the image of God is an important corrective to this tendency.

We may struggle to appreciate the image of God, not only in people who are different from us but also when illness has distorted our patients' bodies and impaired their capacities.[15] As a gastroenterologist, my patients with advanced liver disease come to mind. They are jaundiced and lethargic. Their muscles are wasted and their abdomens protrude with ascites. Their thinking is confused and they may be unable to appreciate the efforts others are making on their behalf. Their condition is sometimes, in part, related to their own unhealthy choices. It's easy to tacitly assume that their physical state and diminished capacities have degraded their value as human beings. Yet the best caregivers see past all of this. They maintain an understanding of the full humanity of their patient—and hence the value of their own work. They learn about the person they're caring for, sometimes from their family, with questions such as, "What does your sister love to do?" or "Tell me what your dad is like." They celebrate even small improvements, and they have the audacity to imagine full restoration of health. They bring a kind and generous outlook to their work and a radical hospitality in their approach to caregiving.[16] They find value in caring for debilitated persons because they are fellow human beings.[17]

The Image of God and the Difficult Patient

Most of us have cared for patients who are hostile, aggressive, threatening, resentful, or erratic. When caring for such people, we must, of course, take measures to protect ourselves and others. There are even times when we must sever our professional or institutional relationship with a patient, no longer providing care to someone who refuses to change their behavior. However, these patients are made in God's likeness as well. When we keep this in mind, it alters our approach. We continue to treat them with respect, even when they do not reciprocate. We listen to their complaints and honestly consider their perspective. We assess whether medical or psychological processes beyond their control are contributing to their behavior and need treatment. We ask about their fears, concerns, past experiences, and assumptions about healthcare, all of which may be driving their maladaptive behavior. We consider whether spiritual factors such as religious struggle or spiritual oppression are at play. We remind them of the image of God by affirming their ability to respect, trust, and appreciate others—including their healthcare team. In all of these ways, faith equips us to use best professional practice in our response to difficult patients. By choosing to do so, we reflect the image of God into the situation, to our own benefit.[a]

[a]Brian E. Lacey et al., "De-escalate Don't Escalate: Essential Steps to Effectively Recognize and Manage the Patient Who Is Angry and Disruptive," *American Journal of Gastroenterology* 118, no. 3 (2023): 386-88, http://doi.org/10.14309/ajg.0000000000002090; Emmet Hirsch, "Lessons from an Angry Patient," *New England Journal of Medicine* 379, no. 7 (2018): 607-9, https://doi.org/10.1056/nejmp1803969.

The idea that all people are fundamentally equal and equally deserving of respect can radically change our relationships with coworkers. Medical culture is hierarchical: some of us give orders that others carry out. We hew to lines of authority, and we commonly seek out the opinion of more experienced colleagues. This beneficial division of healthcare work into many different roles may mistakenly lead to a parallel, unstated ranking of human worth. There is a pecking order that runs from the senior surgeon down to housekeeping, and many of us know colleagues who show little consideration for persons further down the ladder. We stand out from this workplace culture by going out of our way to respect all of our coworkers: learning their names and interests, asking for their insights and opinions, thanking them for their work, and treating them as equals.

Are Christians any different? While all people are made in the image of God, the New Testament highlights that God's Spirit dwells within Christians and renews us according to the image of God who created us (Col 3:9-11). Human brokenness has fractured God's image in each of us; his image is like a shattered mirror that no longer reflects a cohesive likeness. But people recognize and value shards of the mirror that still catch and reflect aspects of God's character, and we all instinctively long to have the mirror pieced together again.[18] God's Spirit is restoring the image of God in us, conforming us to his likeness (Rom 8:29, 2 Cor 3:16-18).

It's through our work, as much as through dedicated times of worship, meditation, and prayer, that we realize the image of God. That's because *being* the image of God and *reflecting* the image of God into the world are two sides of the same coin. When we perceive God's presence at our workplace, we receive his comfort and find joy in our work (Ps 16:11). When we do our work as God would have it, we've more fully become his image, and we gain satisfaction (Ps 17:15; Col 3:8-14; Ps 17:15). As we reflect his love and care outward into others' lives, we accomplish the purpose for which we were made.

GOD'S IMAGE IN HEALTHCARE SETTINGS

The very fact that you've chosen to work in healthcare shows that God's image has shaped your sense of life's purpose. We fulfill our purpose and find satisfaction in our careers as his likeness finds increasing expression in and through us. Let's look at how the image of God informs our approach to our patients and ourselves.

The image of God is present in our patients. Healthcare is privileged work because our patients bear God's likeness. Jesus' image is present in all of our patients, and he said that when we care for lonely, needy, and ill people we are, in some sense, caring for him (Mt 25:34-46). For Mother Teresa, this meant that the sick and disadvantaged persons she cared for were Jesus in distressing disguise.[19]

Although the image of God is fractured in all of us, it can be particularly difficult to perceive in healthcare settings. Patients are focused on their symptoms and healthcare providers are focused on professional performance. Persistent illness can sap patients' dignity, creativity, autonomy, and spirituality. For instance, my malnourished patients often lack the energy to express these elements of personhood. As dementia patients lose their executive function, their humanity can seem to shrink. Some of our patients are angry, confused, incontinent, or unresponsive. It's easy for us to forget that our patients are made in the image of God as that image becomes less and less apparent. And when we're busy or stressed, we may fail to perceive glimpses of God's likeness in others, as I almost did with the young woman I described at the start of this chapter. She, by the way, chose not to return to the physician who had been treating her. She found another specialist near her home who took an interest in her goals and priorities.

The Image of God in the Patient with Dementia

How can we affirm that people who are deeply forgetful, uncommunicative, or unresponsive still bear God's image? We can begin by remembering that human value is not rooted in our ability to remember, reason, or respond. Mutually satisfying interactions with persons with dementia can't rely on these faculties or on our own need for affirmation or thanks. To the extent that such patients are aware of and engaged with the present, we can interact with them about what's happening now and adjust their environment to bring them peace or delight. Physical presence, gentle touch, social or material cues from their earlier life, familiar music, and prayer may all evoke the image of God embedded in them and bring them comfort. At other times, "offering one's presence to a person with dementia means letting go of our need for rational interchanges, direct social cues, logical conclusions. It often means letting go of words altogether and entering entirely into the realm of affect and intuition."[a] If you participate in dementia care, consider reading detailed theological and practical guides that are available.[b]

---

[a] Julie Wolkoff, "Finding God's Image in the World of Dementia," Sefaria, 2017, www .sefaria.org/sheets/90013?lang=bi.

[b] John Swinton, *Dementia: Living in the Memories of God* (Grand Rapids, MI: Eerdmans, 2012); Nancy L. Mace and Peter V. Rabins, *The 36-Hour Day: A Family Guide to Caring for People Who Have Alzheimer's Disease and Other Dementias* (Baltimore: Johns Hopkins University Press, 2021).

The image of God is present in you. The likeness of God is the most valuable personal resource we have. From it springs what we cherish most about ourselves. We fulfill our purpose when the image of God shines brightly from us, and we muddle through life when it is obscured or forgotten. Being God's image doesn't mean that we "play God" at work. Instead, the image of God becomes more and more apparent in our day-to-day lives as we invite his Spirit to work in us and when his character finds expression in our life and work.

> The likeness of God is the most valuable personal resource we have. From it springs what we cherish most about ourselves.

Workplace culture can either facilitate or frustrate that expression. It's difficult to be Christ's image when there are too few workers for the work, or our colleagues devalue patients who are difficult or incapacitated, or financial return is paramount, or incentives discourage us from spending a few extra moments with a patient. In these situations we reflect the image of God when we go against the tide. We can be countercultural agents of change, promoting healthy healthcare structures—or we can find employment in a better workplace.

Because we're made in his image, God's presence is a key personal resource for us. When we recognize God's presence while we're working, we experience his caring concern for us and receive the wisdom we need in real time. Many of this book's exercises are designed to help you experience God's presence while you're at work.

We seek to discover the image of God in our patients. Caring competently for persons includes recognizing the image of God in which they were made. When we perceive elements of God's likeness in our patients and call them out, we affirm the truth about who they are. The image of God gives us and our patients a commonality, a bond that an algorithm or machine can't replace. As we recognize aspects of God's likeness in a patient—especially when that image has been obscured or neglected— we connect with them at a spiritual level, enhance our therapeutic relationship, and increase the satisfaction we get from our work. But uncovering God's image can be like clearing the dust and cobwebs away

from a broken stone to make out its inscription and design. How can we
do that with our patients?

Treat our patients with respect. By treating our patients with gentleness
and consideration, we bear witness to the image of God embedded in
both them and us, and that image becomes easier to perceive. Many times
we acknowledge our patients' worth by exerting ourselves to meet their
medical needs, going the extra mile for them, or serving as their advocate
and guide through the healthcare system. For me, this often means answering their calls promptly, listening to them attentively, taking their
questions seriously, and displaying an unhurried manner. At other times
I acknowledge my patient was made in the image of God by pausing to
ask them about their goals and concerns, or by telling them about the
patience, bravery, persistence, good humor, or strength of character
they've shown in the face of illness. When my patients irritate me, the
knowledge that we both bear God's image leads me to respond with curiosity, not anger. Caring for them this way develops a strong therapeutic
alliance that facilitates their treatment.

Take an interest in our patients as persons. Our patients are more than
their medical conditions. By telling us about their passions, accomplishments, challenges, and loves, they often reveal elements of the image of
God. Oncologist and writer Dr. Al Weir suggests that we daily ask each
of our patients a nonmedical question and tell them one nonmedical
fact about ourselves.[20] I often start a patient interaction by saying, "Tell
me about yourself" or (for returning patients) asking, "What's new in
your life?" Some patients deflect these conversational gambits, but most
enjoy answering. One surgeon I've worked with routinely takes an employment history from his patients, and another leads with "How was
your summer [or spring, fall, or winter]?" Another colleague makes a
point of asking what her patients do for fun. And the best communi-
cators don't leave it there: they ask a follow-up question, such as, "Why
did you go into that line of work?" or "What's the best part of that for
you?" or simply "Can you tell me more?"—getting beyond facts to the
underlying values, emotions, or proclivities of the person. Open-ended
questions (which can't be answered with a simple yes or no) help me

learn what my patients care about and enjoy, how they define themselves in relation to their work, family, or faith, and where they find their
own sense of purpose and significance. These sorts of questions also
help our patients understand that we recognize them as more than an
assembly of body parts or organ systems. In response, they show us
more of themselves. These conversational strategies, which may take
only seconds of time, create a tacit acknowledgment that becomes the
basis for more transparent, productive, and efficient clinical interactions, and better clinical decisions.[21]

Make space for their autonomy and creativity. Our patients were created
to rule. If possible, give them opportunity to express their preferences and
make their own decisions, and encourage them to reengage with their
passions, pleasures, and pastimes.

When approaching treatment options, coach patients through a decision-making process by asking about their goals and concerns. Shared
medical decision-making can empower patients and enhance our own
role as their guide along the healthcare path they are traveling. When your
patient asks a question, look for an unstated worry or goal behind what
they've asked. One simple way to recognize patients' autonomy in the
course of a busy day is to ask, "What would you prefer?" or "What are
your concerns today?"

Help them cope. Perhaps you think that helping patients cope is not
your thing. You are in healthcare to treat disease, not to accommodate it.
But treatment often entails cost, discomfort, risks, and temporary disability. These are realities your patients need to cope with if their treatment
is to succeed. In addition, many of us regularly interact with patients
whose disease process can't be cured. Learning how to successfully cope
with their condition is key to good outcomes for these patients.

Many of our patients are uncomfortable in healthcare settings and wish
they did not need our professional services. We can help them cope with
the process of healthcare by greeting them warmly, learning and remembering nonmedical facts about them, providing a comfortable environment, warming our hands and stethoscopes, addressing their fears,
and not inflicting pain.

A diagnosis can bring with it anxiety, sadness, shame, and loss of hope. Oftentimes we help our patients cope with these feelings by telling them that they will get better. This is particularly important when they are debilitated by their disease and its treatment and may need months to return to health. My patients with severe pancreatitis come to mind: even after leaving the hospital, they may suffer from pain and fatigue, have difficulty eating, lack energy, experience setbacks, and undergo multiple interventional procedures. They often need to be encouraged that the medical marathon they're running has a finish line and that they can look forward to feeling healthy again.

In other cases, though, we best help our patients cope by asking them questions that get at their emotional, social, and spiritual concerns. An oncologist describes how his own diagnosis of colorectal cancer changed his approach to his patients:

> [I used to] talk to patients about the stage of their disease, the science behind the treatments we were going to do, and what we understand about the biology of their disease. My diagnosis has given me a lot more empathy and changed the way I interact with patients. Before we dive into what we are going to do, I ask them: How are you sleeping at night? How is your mood? How did hearing the word "cancer" change things for you?[22]

In place of statements about science and medicine, he now starts with questions that reveal the impact a diagnosis has had on his patients' lives.

Similarly, a urologist finds that his patients make better treatment choices when he asks, "What does this diagnosis mean to you?" before detailing therapeutic options. Their answers often reveal what's important to them—whether it's living as long as possible, or avoiding potential suffering and disability, or dealing with the cost of treatment, or minimizing the impact of their illness on their family. He is then able to address their priorities as he guides them through a decision-making process.[23] When we ask for our patients' perspective, we signal that our interest goes beyond biology and statistics to their individual needs and desires, tacitly recognizing the image of God they bear.

Learn about their spirituality. We humans are spiritual beings. As we'll see later, our spirituality affects our health, and leading secular healthcare organizations advise us to take an interest in our patients' religious practices and spiritual needs. Perceiving the image of God in our patients includes learning about their spirituality. Assessing a patient's spirituality by taking a spiritual history, as outlined in chapter three, is an important first step toward encouraging their spiritual health.

Think differently about our time. In a busy healthcare practice, there may seem to be little time to learn about our patients' lives or to give them the opportunity to express their preferences, concerns, and priorities. Yet treating our patients as more than objects is important, not only for them but also for us. Simple strategies, such as sitting down to talk to a patient at their eye level rather than standing above them, looking at our patient rather than a computer monitor while they're talking, and expressing empathy with sentences that begin with "You," not "I," enhance our communication without requiring more time. Asking open-ended questions and tolerating silence in order to give patients time to respond may lengthen the time we spend with them, although we can often interact with patients this way while we're simultaneously doing something else: moving through a physical exam or administering a medication, for instance. Matters sometimes emerge from such interactions that require additional conversation and care, extending the time required. These minutes are not time wasted. They are moments that can lead us directly to the crux of who our patient is and what they need. In my experience, an initial investment of time in the care of a patient can establish mutual trust and unearth hidden issues from the start, enhancing our communication, saving time in the long run, and resulting in better outcomes. Holistic care can be efficient care.

Is it worth it? Perhaps you're thinking that work is easier when we ignore the image of God embedded in our patients and ourselves and simply focus on medical tasks. This may at times be true, and sometimes the volume of work or our patients' acute needs leave us no

Holistic care can be efficient care.

choice. But there is a tradeoff involved: when we treat our patients as commodities, we gradually stray from our purpose and cheat ourselves of satisfaction. An analogy may help. Gems and gravel are both rocks, but they differ in value, and we treat them differently. Our patients are valuable because they are image bearers. We healthcare professionals are jewelers, but it's easy to lose sight of the image of God and come to believe that we're shoveling gravel. This doesn't serve our patients well, and when we're blind to the unique nature of people, we miss out on much of the significance of our work.

FOR REFLECTION

1. Our overarching purpose as human beings is to be God's image and reflect his image into the world. To what extent is a healthcare career fulfilling or hindering your purpose?

2. Can you think of a patient you initially viewed as a medical problem but later thought of as a child of God? What triggered the change in your perspective?

3. The United States Surgeon General writes, "Burnout is characterized by a high degree of emotional exhaustion and depersonalization (i.e., cynicism) and a low sense of personal accomplishment at work."[24] Overwork, lack of rest, the burden of others' suffering, an inequitable work culture, moral injury or posttraumatic stress, depression, and lack of spiritual refreshment may all contribute. Burned out healthcare workers have lost touch with the purpose and meaning of their work and may be less likely to perceive the image of God in their patients or in themselves. What steps might be necessary to recover this perception?

4. Describe practical ways you can perceive elements of the image of God in your patients without much lengthening the time you spend with them. Review the practical suggestions in the last half of this chapter and adapt them to your own situation.

IT'S YOUR TURN

Paying for a gym membership doesn't get you into better physical shape. You have to use the gym. In the same way, ideas from this chapter will not enhance your professional satisfaction unless you put them into practice. Pick one of the following exercises and practice it this week:

1. While at work, practice being the image of God. This might mean silently humming a worship song while you log on to a workstation, stand in line at the cafeteria, or clean your hands between patients—your spirit communing for a moment with God's Spirit. It might involve going above and beyond what's required for one of your patients, showing consideration to someone who doesn't seem to deserve it, or finding gracious and encouraging ways to interact with people. These actions remind you that your connection to God—not your work—defines who you are.

2. Before each patient encounter, pray silently for a few seconds. Ask God to help you perceive his image in your next patient and to care for them with ingenuity and skill.

3. Affirm that your patients are image bearers, even if they have no faith or a faith that is different from yours. Use one or more of the methods described in this chapter: show respect, take an interest in them as persons, acknowledge their autonomy, encourage their creativity, help them cope, validate their strengths, learn about their spirituality. For starters, you could try asking every patient you care for this week a nonmedical question and follow up with an additional question that goes beyond facts to their perceptions, preferences, or values.

2

Body

I HAVE A FRIEND, A MISSIONARY SURGEON, who sees little ultimate value in meeting patients' physical needs. Although she spent a decade in medical school and surgical training and now spends most of her waking hours practicing surgery, she says, "If I fix my patient's physical problem, but they don't become a follower of Jesus, I've left them worse off than when they first came to see me." She reasons that her patients will all die sooner or later, but their souls will live on for eternity. The salvation of their souls is therefore infinitely more important than their physical health. In marketing terms, her surgical skills are a hook that lands sick, injured, or disabled people in her hospital, where they can hear the gospel. She has curtailed her operating room schedule so that she can spend more time counseling and praying with patients.

I also know Christians practicing in secular contexts who, like my friend, believe that souls are the only things that matter in the long run. However, proselytizing is counter to the ethos of their patients and the secular healthcare institutions in which they work. Lobbying their patients to convert would violate the spirit of their employment, and they might be criticized or disciplined if they did so. Since evangelism in the hospital and clinic is not appropriate, they shy away from any explicit consideration of spirituality during their patient interactions, and they conclude that their healthcare work has little or no eternal value. Their faith informs their practice only insofar as it makes them exemplars of ethical standards, such as placing the patient's needs first, that are also broadly accepted by their colleagues.

I think that my surgeon friend's desire to care for souls is admirable. And I empathize with my colleagues who, practicing in secular settings, see little or no overarching significance in their healthcare work. However, the belief these people share that the care of bodies has no everlasting value is mistaken. Oftentimes this belief is based on the assumption, expressed by Gnostic philosophers in the centuries after Jesus' death, that the body is temporary and of dubious value, and salvation belongs to the soul alone. In this view, bodies are at best disposable biological shells, having little to do with our immaterial inner selves. But this supposition doesn't account for a biblical view of personhood, the prominent role of healing in Jesus' own ministry, or how the Bible describes salvation.

Scripture repeatedly instructs believers to address the practical needs of the people around them.[1] Those needs matter because we humans are bodies. Our physicality is not an optional or temporary part of us.

Throughout this book we'll consider the relevance of bodies to the eternal scheme of things. In this chapter, we'll look at the biblical evidence that the human body is good and that our physicality is a necessary dimension of our humanity, both now and in the hereafter. We'll also begin to explore why Jesus often chose to heal people, and why we (like him) choose to spend our time caring for bodies that are destined to die. The Bible's teaching about these topics might surprise you—and it will shape your understanding of your work.

THE BODY IS GOOD AND ESSENTIAL TO OUR IDENTITY

The Gnostic heresy emerged during the first centuries after Jesus' death and resurrection. The Gnostics taught that the physical world and the human body were corrupt and temporary.[2] According to them, spirit was good and body was bad. The early church fathers rejected this teaching. They followed the Judeo-Christian Scriptures, which teach that the physical world in general, and the human body in particular, are God's excellent and enduring creation.

The Genesis account depicts God designing the human body and giving it life: "Then the Lord God formed a man from the dust of the ground and breathed into his nostrils the breath of life, and the man became a living being" (Gen 2:7). Adam and Eve were created from the earth's elements and brought to life as personal, biological beings.[3] God didn't create their souls and spirits first and then install them into bodies later on. They were bodies from the start.[4] Their physicality was intrinsic to their identity and essential to their being.

Adam and Eve were made before brokenness entered the human experience, and God declared them, like all of his creation, good (Gen 1:31). The Hebrew word for "good" can encompass aesthetic, emotional, ethical, and moral connotations.[5] In the immediate context of Genesis 1, it implies the capacity to fulfill the purpose for which we were made.[6] The human body was designed by God, the master Creator, who does all things well.

God continues to create bodies today. Psalm 139, which describes the prenatal development of King David, shows that God kept making humans long after Adam and Eve. As with Adam, the account again starts with David's body, which was "woven together" from the elements of earth. Using his parents' genetic codes, God formed David's body in utero, and David says that his body was wonderfully made. This holds true for all of us. God knows our bodies from their inception, before we know ourselves, and he superintends the development of each fetus. God creates good things—even after the fall described in Genesis 3, and despite the imperfections and illnesses we suffer from, our bodies are good.

What's more, Jesus became a human body. John, writing about him, says, "The Word became flesh and made his dwelling among us" (Jn 1:14; see also 1 Jn 1:1-2). Jesus, like you and I, existed physically. Since he lived a blameless life (1 Pet 2:22), we can conclude that the human body is not intrinsically evil. Furthermore, we can again conclude that physicality is an essential dimension of human beings. In order to be human, Jesus had to enter his creation as a biological person, not a ghost. Far from being optional, his body played an integral role in his mission: we read in the New Testament that he "'bore our sins' in his body on the cross" (1 Pet 2:24), and that he reconciled us to God "in his body

> Physicality is an essential dimension of human beings. In order to be human, Jesus had to enter his creation as a biological person, not a ghost.

of flesh by his death" (Col 1:22 ESV). During Communion we commemorate his body broken for us.

The resurrected Jesus is a body. When he first appears to his disciples after his death and resurrection, they are "startled and frightened, thinking they saw a ghost" (Lk 24:37). Jesus responds, "It is I myself! Touch me and see; a ghost does not have flesh and bones, as you see I have" (Lk 24:39). He then eats food in their presence (Lk 24:41-43). The food doesn't drop through him to the floor; it remains in his stomach. Later, when Jesus leaves his disciples and ascends into heaven, he doesn't abandon his body here on earth. He is "taken up before their very eyes, and a cloud hid him from their sight" (Acts 1:9). At his future second coming, Jesus will return physically (Acts 1:11). His body is enduring evidence of his humanity.

God's Spirit inhabits each Christian's body. Urging the Corinthian Christians to avoid sexual promiscuity, Paul writes, "Do you not know that your bodies are temples of the Holy Spirit, who is in you, whom you have received from God?" (1 Cor 6:19). A temple is a place where God is present and where people worship. It is not an evil place. God's Spirit dwells in our bodies—in our material selves. This means that God does not deal with us only as spirits. He is present in our physicality. As temples, our bodies have spiritual significance. They are "claimed by God, loved by God, and can respond to God."[7] We worship God not by leaving our bodies but with our bodies.

Faith is not merely intellectual assent to a set of beliefs. It is a bodily commitment. When God established a binding relationship with Abraham and his descendants, he required in return that they "walk before me faithfully" (Gen 17:1). Walking, of course, is a bodily activity, and throughout the Bible it is used as shorthand for our behavior over time (Gen 17:1-2; see also Jn 8:12, 11:9; Gal 5:16, 25; 1 Jn 1:6-7; 2 Jn 1:6; 3 Jn 1:4; Rev 3:4). To walk faithfully is to routinely act in ways consistent with our allegiance to God. For Christians, the presence of God's Spirit within us gives us a responsibility to honor him with our bodily choices and physical actions. The commitment Abraham and his male descendants made to God was

> We worship God not by leaving our bodies but with our bodies.

embodied by a physical alteration—circumcision—which God called "my covenant in your flesh" (Gen 17:13). Circumcision was bodily evidence of identification and allegiance. For Christians, the physical act of baptism has similar significance. It is a demonstration that our whole selves have been buried and raised with Jesus (Gen 17:13; see also Rom 6:4-7).[8]

Death is not the end of our bodies. In his letter to the Philippians, Paul writes, "Our citizenship is in heaven. And we eagerly await a Savior from there, the Lord Jesus Christ, who, by the power that enables him to bring everything under his control, will transform our lowly bodies so that they will be like his glorious body" (Phil 3:20-21). For us as for Jesus, the body is an enduring dimension of being human. We don't leave our anatomy behind forever when we die. Jesus will reconstitute our bodies, changing them into the sort of body he already has. The Christian concept of resurrection is more than a metaphor: it's the actual re-creation of a body that died, transformed and animated in new ways.[9] Jesus' resurrected body bears the scars of his physical suffering. Those scars demonstrate a continuity of self from mortal life through to resurrection, and indicate that temporal, material events have eternal significance. We will be resurrected as individuals, and marks of our physical suffering or disability might persist in our resurrected selves also.[10] Nevertheless, our resurrection bodies will be glorious, and we will be healthy.

We are bodies. Bodies are not temporary housing, problems to be overcome, or distractions from our better selves. However, the word *flesh* sometimes has negative connotations in the Pauline epistles, which can lead to confusion about the goodness of the human body. Paul often uses this word to refer not to our physicality but to our unredeemed nature, opposed to God and prone to self-deception and self-destruction.[11] He nowhere contradicts Scripture's depiction of the body as God's good creation or asserts that the physical body is immoral.

SALVATION IS CORPOREAL

If you're like me, you grew up with images of heaven as a place where winged human spirits float through the air and sit on the clouds. This is not a biblical view of the hereafter. In Christ's future, fully realized kingdom, we will have resurrected bodies. We will eat, work, laugh, and love. Theologian Christoffer Grundmann asserts that "redemption is corporeal," following Scripture, which refers to the physical aspect of salvation as "the redemption of our bodies" (Rom 8:23).[12] Our salvation, which begins when we accept Jesus' sacrifice for us and give him our allegiance, will not be complete until we become resurrected bodies.[13] The bodily dimension of salvation helps explain why healing figured prominently in the ministry of Jesus.

When Jesus visited communities, he rescued human spirits by casting out demons, restored bodies by healing, and saved souls by preaching repentance.[14] Healing was an essential element of his work that demonstrated his intention to redeem whole people. By healing sickness and disability, Jesus was showing the importance of bodily restoration as an element of salvation, up to and including raising people from the dead (Jn 11). The healings he performed were harbingers of the complete and permanent healing Christians will experience at his second coming.

When we healthcare professionals heal bodies, we don't perfect them. Our restorative powers are at a quite modest level compared to the future transformation Scripture tells us about. Yet the healing we can accomplish is a divine gift to our patients. It too is a harbinger of the transformation we will experience when heaven comes down to earth (Rev 21:1-2). "By caring for others now, Christian healthcare workers seek to honor the goodness of our bodies and anticipate future resurrection."[15]

What About People Who Are Not Physically Healed?

We are destined to die. Death is often painful, untimely, and tragic. Some of us bear chronic medical conditions that remind us of our limitations and our mortality. Yet David writes that God "heals all your diseases" (Ps 103:3). Why, if our bodies are good and Jesus saves whole persons, not just souls, are we still susceptible to illness and death?

One answer is that Jesus has won victory over sickness and death, but his transforming work in us and throughout his creation is not yet complete. His kingdom continues to break into the world, but the world in general and our bodies in particular are still marred by the curses of Genesis 3. Like all of creation, we're still in "bondage to decay" (Rom 8:21). Christ-followers are in the process of becoming more like Jesus, a process that will not be complete until our resurrection. In the meantime, the tremendous advances in health-care over the past century are evidence of God's common grace given to all people. Biblical statements such as "the prayer offered in faith will make the sick person well; the Lord will raise them up" (Jas 5:15) are general statements of what we can expect in the ordinary course of things. They are not blanket assurances that we will always recover from illness or never die.

Despite the promise of future renewal, suffering and death can seem inexplicable in a world governed by an all-powerful, all-loving God. How we can best respond to that dilemma in the here and now is the subject of the third section of this book.

BURNOUT

For years I would cover emergency gastrointestinal endoscopy services as an attending physician for a week at a time. I enjoyed taking care of emergencies and working with the fellow, training to be a specialist, who was also assigned to the service. When it was busy I would get little sleep, often for several days in a row. As time went by, I found it increasingly difficult to respond to two a.m. telephone calls night after night. The work was becoming exhausting, but I didn't realize the impact fatigue was having on me until one of our fellows gave me a poor review after we spent a week working together. They said that I was technically proficient but lacked empathy.

It's easy to fall into one of two opposite and incorrect ways of thinking about our bodies and their limitations. On the one hand, we can go through life believing that the body is expendable and temporary and that only our immaterial selves matter. This approach to life and health focuses on intangible realities. It makes us inattentive to our body's limits, functions, and needs, impairing our health. In this way of thinking, we take care of ourselves by ignoring, exploiting, or denying our bodies. It was this view that I had lapsed into while covering emergency endoscopy for a week at a time. Unwilling to recognize my need for rest, I was blind to the impact fatigue was having on my approach to my patients and colleagues. My humanity, and the human elements of my work, were suffering.

On the other hand, we can live as though we are no more than bodies. This approach to life and health focuses only on physical realities. It leads us to confuse bodily health and comfort with meaning and purpose, and the absence of physical difficulties with thriving. In this way of thinking, we take care of ourselves by exercising or pampering our bodies. Exercise is good, naps are restorative, and satisfying our bodily appetites is both necessary and enjoyable—but when these become our principal motivations in life, we're missing purposes beyond ourselves and our spirits may atrophy.

In the Christian understanding there is a middle way between these two extremes. Life is more than our biology, but our being, purpose, and significance are embedded in our bodies. Without our bodies we do not exist in space and time. We are a beautiful combination of flesh and bone, soul and spirit. We thrive when we enjoy each of these dimensions of personhood and meet each of their needs. We suffer when we either focus mainly on our bodies or ignore them.

Our bodies are good and essential elements of our humanity. We need rest, balanced nutrition, exercise, and recreation. Yet our professional careers will often take as much time and energy from us as we're willing to give, even when this causes us to skimp on what our bodies need and jeopardize our own well-being. Both our healthcare practices and our personal lives suffer when we're out of balance physically: we become emotionally fragile, prone to anger, less empathetic, less interested in others, and less attentive, resilient, insightful, and creative. Overwork and fatigue make me impatient and critical of my team members. When I find myself becoming angry at work, I've learned to stop and examine my own emotional and physical health.

The quality of our work easily degrades when there is too much of it. A nurse who is now routinely working sixteen-hour shifts told me she is concerned that fatigue is leading to medical errors on her hospital unit. In my own field, the quality of colonoscopies decreases as workloads

> Life is more than our biology, but our being, purpose, and significance are embedded in our bodies. Without our bodies we do not exist in space and time.

increase and is worst at the end of the workweek.[16] Our job satisfaction and overall health suffer when we don't have sufficient time away from clinical responsibilities. A colleague recently told me, "Medicine is high stakes, and that's a lot to bear all the time." Even when she isn't at work, she can rarely escape from the medical record in-basket for more than a few waking hours. But we all need time off. Our blood pressure and stress hormone levels decrease when we're on holiday, and the risk of myocardial infarction and death is lower in persons who take regular vacations.[17] The Japanese word *karoshi* refers to sudden death associated with too much work or occupational stress, and a related word refers to occupation-related suicide.[18] Paradoxically, we need limits on our work hours and time away from healthcare to have a long, healthy, and satisfying healthcare career.

The systems we work in should respect our God-given needs and limitations. If our workplace culture is unhealthy, we can advocate for change or find a better system to work in. I earlier mentioned the poor review I received while covering emergency endoscopy; after that episode, we staffed emergency services differently so that there were regularly scheduled off-call rest hours throughout the week. Are you a leader in your hospital, office, or medical practice? Prioritize the physical well-being of your colleagues and employees.

WHY BOTHER CARING FOR BODIES?

We healthcare workers spend our careers caring for human bodies. Yet we know that our work doesn't prevent the inevitability of death. Why, then, do we invest our time and energy in restoring physical health? Is there any everlasting value in healing human bodies? After two chapters we have some answers:

Healthcare work is good, God-appointed work. God gave Adam and Eve the work of caring for the world he created. By restoring people's health, we're doing the same work, as God's emissaries in the here and now. When we treat bodies, we're carrying out the stewardship mandate of Genesis 1: tending God's creation, reflecting his love and care into the lives of people, fulfilling the purpose for which we were made.

This means that we rightly draw satisfaction from working to mend human bodies. We can find deep fulfillment from using our skills to bend creation toward healing. Contentment comes from doing what God has gifted and intended us to do, with care and excellence, while leaving the results up to him. We strive for good patient outcomes, and they are rewarding—they're the cherry, whipped cream, and chocolate sauce on top of the ice cream sundae—but our satisfaction is rooted in the work itself.

Bodies are good and eternal elements of our identity. Our physicality is an essential dimension of who we are. What's more, the meaning and purpose of life are embedded in our bodies, and we enable patients to pursue their purpose by addressing their physical ailments. Medical care touches the enduring nature of human beings and can have everlasting echoes in their lives.

Jesus healed bodies. In the Gospel accounts, people often come to Jesus for help with their health problems. Jesus typically addresses their felt need—their "chief complaint"—by healing them, whether or not they subsequently choose to praise God (Lk 17:11-19). Similarly, people come to us with their afflictions, and we work hard to cure or ease these problems, regardless of their views about spirituality, or whether their relationship with God will subsequently be renewed. As we care for bodily needs, with excellence, we bring Christ's good gift of health to people. Their healing, as we'll see in chapter 11, is for them a close encounter with his kingdom.

Medicine casts a spiritual shadow. As we'll see in the next chapter, bodily illness and healing have ramifications for the soul and spirit. The experience of sickness and healing brings life's spiritual realities into focus for many patients. Physical problems can distort our entire being, and spiritual renewal can accompany bodily healing. There are time-efficient and context-appropriate ways to connect to this reality at the point of care. Doing so aligns us with our purpose and brings fulfillment.

FOR REFLECTION

1. Do you agree that the body is good? If you disagree on some points, review and discuss the relevant Bible passages referenced in this chapter.

2. Could the belief that the body is good and essential to our identity affect the fulfillment you derive from working in healthcare? Consider the summary points at the conclusion of this chapter.

3. Our bodies are temples of the Holy Spirit, but it's often easy to neglect them when life gets busy. Are there warning signs in your own life that you are skimping on your bodily needs? What attention does your body require? How can you start addressing it this week?

IT'S YOUR TURN

1. Taking care of your own body can enhance your ability to care for others and the satisfaction you get from work. Identify one thing you can do this week to better meet your bodily needs. It might be sleep, exercise, massage, investing in comfortable shoes, scheduling a medical or dental checkup, buying a better mattress, looking for a new job with better hours, altering your diet, or something else.

2. Our day-to-day work with bodies is good, God-appointed work. God is working in your patients' lives, and you are a part of what he is doing. Before you step into each patient encounter this week, align yourself with him by offering a brief prayer just before you walk through the door and greet your next patient. Invite God to use you—your professional skills and personal manner—to bring healing to them.

3

Soul and Spirit

I SOMETIMES SEE PATIENTS with unrelenting abdominal pain that has come on months or years after gallbladder surgery. Often the pain and its treatment have dramatically altered their lives. One such patient had given up her job because she could no longer concentrate on her work. The pain medications she was taking had helped initially, but over time they had made her more sensitive to the pain, which could rise to intolerable levels when she ate, sat in a chair or car, or carried laundry upstairs. She became housebound, and her social circle shrank. She was alone and idle much of the time. She fell into depression and began taking medication for that as well.

In her case, I identified and treated a cluster of nerve endings that were the root cause of her pain. When she returned to see me a month later, she seemed like a different person. She was smiling and talkative. "I can live again," she said. "Things aren't perfect, but I can eat without worrying about the pain. I've been taking walks, seeing friends and going out with my husband. It would be great to go back to work. Thank you!" Her long-afflicted soul and spirit, once closeted, were starting to flourish again. I told her that I had been praying for her and that I too was thankful she was better.

For me, patients like this are memorable because a medical intervention released their whole self from the constraints of disease. The soul and the spirit are essential dimensions of human beings. They may be affected by bodily illness, and they can in turn influence physical health.

It's when we restore bodies, souls, and spirits—whole persons—that we find the greatest significance in healthcare work. Yet many of us feel uncomfortable talking with our patients about their souls and spirits, and unsure how we would go about such conversations. In this chapter we'll begin by considering what the soul and the spirit are. We'll then look at the evidence that spirituality and physical health are related. Finally, we'll describe how to take a spiritual history—a broadly accepted assessment that helps us perceive the spiritual dimension of our work.

WHAT ARE SOUL AND SPIRIT?

In the Bible's original languages there are several words translated as "soul" and "spirit." These terms usually refer to nonanatomic aspects of ourselves, and they have broad semantic ranges, with overlapping, occasionally physical meanings.[1] This linguistic overlap tells us that a human is body, soul, and spirit tightly knit together into a unified being. We can't actually separate these aspects of personhood from each other. If I asked you to remove all the white threads from my white, blue, and red shirt, I wouldn't have a shirt by the time you were done! N. T. Wright says that these terms each refer to "the *whole* human being *seen from one angle*."[2] Although it's impossible for us to dissect the human body, soul, and spirit away from each other, some Bible passages do distinguish between them.[3] Considering the distinctive emphases of the words *soul* and *spirit*—words that, for our purposes, encompass our psychology and our capacity to relate on a transcendent, spiritual plane—can help us understand the full dimensionality of human beings, and the role our immaterial selves play in sickness and health.

Soul is shorthand for the embodied life of each human being. It is the "vital spark that animates us in the present life."[4] It is our living being, driving our choices and actions.[5] The word *psychology* derives from *psychē*, the Greek word for "soul," and refers to the study of mind and behavior. The soul encompasses our mind, will, desires, emotions, ambitions, and personality.[6] Your soul gets you out of bed in the morning, and it motivates you throughout the day. It is an immaterial expression of your individuality.

The human spirit is that dimension of us that relates to God.[7] Our spirits transcend (or reach beyond) ourselves and the visible world around us to relate to other spirits. They give us a deep connection to the divine—a kinship—so much so that we can be one with God (1 Cor 6:17). He can commune with us, indwell us, speak to us, and lead us (Rom 8:14-16). People who don't believe in God often report spiritual experiences, which they may describe as a connection to the world or universe. Spiritual experiences of both religious and nonreligious people are characterized by a sense of relationship and wonder, and often cause feelings of awe, "small self," and humility.[8] All people have spirits, and the Bible attests to our ability to communicate with other spirits via a spiritual dimension of reality that, so far as we know, is not physical.[9] Spirituality is a relational plane, and our important relationships often include a spiritual bond.[10] The relational nature of our spirits informs our choices and behavior.[11]

In modern cultures our connection to spiritual reality can fade. Our spirits can atrophy, and we can move through our days largely oblivious to the spiritual dimension of life. Yet our inability to perceive spiritual reality doesn't invalidate its existence. Instead, it suggests we may be suffering from a sort of spiritual blindness. It's as though we've lost one of our senses or are seeing the world in black-and-white.[12] However, there are many examples of persons who are living in full color, alert both to God and to the spirits of other people.

Perhaps, like me, you find that when you exercise your spirituality through prayer and Scripture reading, you are more likely to sense God's direction at key moments during your workday. During my medical training I knew a laboratory scientist who would occasionally awaken in the middle of the night with a compelling need to pray for a stranger. He sometimes found out weeks or months later who the person was and what had happened to them. Another colleague, who grew up in an African culture, was walking home from work one evening and felt the urge to walk past her house and go

> Our inability to perceive spiritual reality doesn't invalidate its existence. Instead, it suggests we may be suffering from a sort of spiritual blindness.

farther down the sidewalk to visit the home of a coworker. She found her friend preparing to commit suicide. When I was a boy my great-grandmother, an immigrant from the old world, visited me in my dreams one night to say goodbye. I was not surprised when, at breakfast the next morning, my father told our family that she had died during the night. These are all examples that point to spiritual reality.

We can exercise our spirituality like we exercise our bodies. For Christians, prayer, worship, and Scripture are on-ramps to the spiritual and means of developing spiritual alertness and effectiveness. We better perceive the spiritual dimension of work and life as we become increasingly aware of God's presence in our workplaces.

SOULS, SPIRITS, AND BODILY HEALTH

This side of the grave, a human being is a single, inseparable combination of the material and the immaterial, of body, soul, and spirit.[13] Each aspect affects the others: soul and spirit leave footprints on the body, and vice versa. This is illustrated in a biblical story about the prophet Elijah.

In this account, Elijah has just had a face-off with the prophets of the idol Baal, capping years of conflict and defeating them in a dramatic encounter on a mountaintop. You might think that Elijah would be exhilarated by this victory, but the wicked queen Jezebel reacts furiously, vowing to kill him. Elijah responds by running for his life. Along the way he leaves a trusted companion behind and flees into the wilderness alone. Spent, he sits down under a tree and prays, "I have had enough, LORD. . . . Take my life; I am no better than my ancestors" (1 Kings 19:4).

Elijah is burnt out. His success has exhausted him, and Jezebel's threat is one challenge too far. His soul is sick: he feels unable to go on, he is driven by fear and ready to die, and he has lost sight of the significance of his work. His spirit is likewise suffering: he is alone, out of touch with others and out of sync with God. Previously he's had a robust relationship with God, from whom he receives direction (see, e.g., 1 Kings 17:2, 8, 22), but now his prayer is a declaration of his exhaustion, with no perception of a divine response. He is at the end of his rope. He falls asleep, and we might wonder whether he will ever wake up.

God sends an angel to Elijah, rousing him and giving him bread and water. His body has been suffering the physical effects of his psychological and spiritual crisis. His mountaintop victory and his flight into the wilderness have left him dehydrated and acutely malnourished. God attends first to his needs for food, drink, and rest. God feeds him repeatedly: Elijah's physical debility takes time to heal.[14]

Restored physically, Elijah is once more able to hear and respond to God. He travels to Mount Horeb, "the mountain of God," where God twice asks him an open-ended question: "What are you doing here, Elijah?" (1 Kings 19:9, 13). God takes Elijah's history of present illness, listening as he pours out his story of defeat and isolation. God then restores Elijah's spirit by showing him how to appreciate God's presence, not in dramatic events but in the silence that follows. Finally, he restores Elijah's soul by correcting his misperceptions. He is not alone: there are thousands of other people in Israel who are faithful to God. Nor is his work finished: Elijah has specific tasks to accomplish, successors to appoint and mentor who will carry on the work. Renewed in body, soul, and spirit, Elijah goes on (1 Kings 19:6-18).

Elijah's story demonstrates the interconnectedness of body, soul, and spirit health, but it is only one example. A serious affliction of our material or immaterial selves can sap the other aspects of personhood. Many of us have cared for patients whose anger, sorrow, or loneliness led them to neglect their physical health until they were forced to seek medical care. Another example is posttraumatic stress, which may be caused by psychological trauma and results in bodily hyperarousal. The resulting physiologic changes can manifest as physical ailments years after the trauma occurred.[15] In my own field of medicine, chronic abdominal pain has been associated with prior psychological or physical abuse in some patients. Bodily interventions such as structured physical exercises may help patients recover from the psychological effects of traumatic stress.[16]

When we treat a patient's physical ailment, we may bring them to a point where their spirit is able and interested in engaging with God. Patients such as the one I described at the start of this chapter, who was suffering from chronic pain, may live in darkness because of their illness:

their world has narrowed to the four windowless walls of their ailment, and their debility has extinguished their hope. When they meet a loving healthcare team, it's as though a glimmer of light has entered their reality. When their health starts to improve, it's as though a window has been opened. Their souls and spirits revive.

Alternatively, our immaterial selves can mitigate the consequences of sickness. Consider people you've known who had strong spiritual and social resources and how these contributed to their recovery from an illness. Interventions directed at the soul can alter our anatomy: psychological therapies for chronic pain can lead to changes in the volume and function of certain regions of the brain.[17]

SPIRITUALITY AND HEALTH OUTCOMES

The concept that our will, emotions, and desires are linked to our physical health may be familiar, but you may be surprised to learn that spirituality also relates to health. Scientific research supports a link between spirituality and a number of important health outcomes:[18]

Religious activity is associated with decreased mortality. Studies from around the world demonstrate decreases in mortality rates ranging from 20 to 40 percent among people who regularly attend religious services compared to those who never attend.[19] These studies analyzed large cohorts of generally healthy people who completed questionnaires and were then followed for a period of years. This mortality benefit is associated with attendance at religious services, not simply religious affiliation.[20] This literature shows that participating regularly in the life of a community of faith is associated with better health.

Religious people tend to engage in healthy behaviors and have strong social networks. In one study, these and other observable factors accounted for only about two-thirds of the mortality improvement religiously active people enjoy.[21] The same group of researchers has subsequently reported associations between spiritually motivated forgiveness of others and well-being, spirituality and lower rates of "death from despair" among healthcare workers, a lower chance of developing hypertension over time in religiously active persons, and lower mortality over time in women who practice gratitude.[22] It's not yet clear whether the physical and mental health benefits that are associated with regular participation in a religious community accrue with virtual or online attendance.

Faith helps patients cope with illness. Persons with chronic or life-threatening illnesses are better able to cope with their condition if faith is a part of their life. This is a consistent finding across many medical studies involving patients with various diseases.[23] Persons of faith believe there is a God who determines life's meaning and significance, as well as their physical circumstances. Without faith, people may think these elements are disconnected or that their bodily health is all-determining. They may feel that they are caught in the machinery of their physical suffering, especially when medical solutions fall short.[24]

Spiritual distress is associated with mortality.[25] Some patients with serious or chronic diseases experience spiritual turmoil related to their illness, a condition called "spiritual distress" or "religious struggle." They answer yes to questions such as, "Do you feel God has abandoned you?" "Do you think God is punishing you?" or "Do you think the devil made this happen to you?"[26] Spiritual distress is common in patients assessed by chaplains.[27] In one study, patients experiencing spiritual distress had increased two-year mortality rates compared to matched control patients without spiritual distress.[28] Spiritual distress has also been associated with psychological distress and lower quality of life in palliative care patients and survivors of serious illness. A study of a national sample of American adults found robust links between religious struggle and psychological distress, depression, and anxiety.[29]

Treatment implications. Emerging research suggests that spiritual interventions can have positive impacts on overall health. For instance, the practice of gratitude is associated with improved medical outcomes, and faith-based cognitive-behavioral therapy—which incorporates elements of the patient's own spirituality into their treatment—is more effective than standard cognitive-behavioral therapy for the treatment of psychiatric disease.[30] The available data seem to justify sensitively assessing patients' spiritual health, addressing issues such as spiritual distress, and incorporating spiritual considerations into overall treatment plans.

BEST-PRACTICE GUIDELINES

The data we've reviewed don't prove that God exists or that any particular religion is true but do lead to the conclusion that robust spirituality has health benefits. Because these research findings are not dependent on the truth of religion, they are broadly applicable in medical contexts where there is no consensus about faith—as in the secular situations where many of us practice. They strongly support a holistic approach to our patients. Assessing spirituality and encouraging spiritual health are therefore best practices in healthcare, and the ability to understand a patient's spirituality is considered a cultural competence of healthcare professionals.[31] As shown in the sidebar "Professional Guidelines Encourage Us to Assess Our Patients' Spirituality," authoritative secular guidelines from well-respected sources encourage us to learn about our patients' spirituality.

Professional Guidelines Encourage Us to Assess Our Patients' Spirituality

The American Association of Medical Colleges' learning objectives for medical students include having the ability to elicit a spiritual history, understanding that the spiritual dimension of people's lives is an avenue for compassionate caregiving, and knowing the research data on the impact of spirituality on health.[a]

The Joint Commission, the leading organization credentialing healthcare facilities across the United States, advises practitioners to conduct a spiritual assessment, at a minimum exploring the patient's denomination or faith tradition, their significant spiritual beliefs, and their important spiritual practices.[b]

The British General Medical Council sets standards for medical practice in the United Kingdom. It states, "In assessing a patient's conditions and taking a history, you should take account of spiritual, religious, social and cultural factors, as well as their clinical history and symptoms."[c]

The International Council of Nurses advises, "The nurse promotes an environment in which the human rights, values, customs and spiritual beliefs of the individual, family and community are respected."[d]

NANDA International, the world's leading nursing diagnosis association, recognizes "impaired religiosity," "readiness for enhanced religiosity," "spiritual distress," and "risk for spiritual distress" as nursing diagnoses meriting treatment plans.[e]

The World Health Organization recommends that healthcare workers and organizations provide "access to social, emotional and spiritual support for patients and their families."[f]

Citations a-f also appear in the Saline Process Witness Training curriculum, version 1.4.

[a]Medical School Objectives Project, *Contemporary Issues in Medicine: Communication in Medicine* (Washington, DC: American Association of Medical Colleges, 1999), https://repository.library.georgetown.edu/handle/10822/927531; see also Christina M. Puchalski, "Spirituality and Medicine: Curricula in Medical Education," *Journal of Cancer Education* 21, no. 1 (2006): 14-18, https://pubmed.ncbi.nlm.nih.gov/16918282/.

[b]David R. Hodge, "A Template for Spiritual Assessment: A Review of the JCAHO Requirements and Guidelines for Implementation," *Social Work* 51, no. 4 (2006): 317-26, http://doi.org/10.1093/sw/51.4.317.

[c]British General Medical Council, "Personal Beliefs and Medical Practice," updated December 2024, www.gmc-uk.org/professional-standards/professional-standards -for-doctors/personal-beliefs-and-medical-practice.

[d]International Council of Nurses, "Code of Ethics for Nurses," revised 2021, www.icn .ch/sites/default/files/2023-06/ICN_Code-of-Ethics_EN_Web.pdf.

[e]NANDA International, *Nursing Diagnoses: Definitions and Classification 2021–2023* (Thieme, 2021), 457-62.

[f]World Health Organization, *People-Centred Health Care: A Policy Framework* (Geneva: World Health Organization, 2007), 12.

TAKING A SPIRITUAL HISTORY

Our material and immaterial selves are woven together and strongly influence each other. Seeing our patients in three dimensions—as biological, psychological, and spiritual beings—can make us better caregivers and deepen the satisfaction we derive from our work. But, in practical terms, how can we perceive our patients' spirituality and find fulfillment in encouraging spiritual health in the middle of a busy healthcare practice? Oftentimes it starts with taking a spiritual history.

Spiritual history-taking consists of asking clinically relevant questions about faith during a patient evaluation. It generally fits most naturally with the social history portion of a patient interview and can become an unapologetic part of your patient assessment—whether you are a doctor, nurse, dentist, emergency medical technician, therapist, or other healthcare professional. There are a number of standard approaches to the spiritual history that have been described in the medical literature, two of which are shown in the sidebar "Two Spiritual History Methods."[32]

Two Spiritual History Methods

FICA, an acronym for faith, importance and influence, community, and address in care, is a common structure for spiritual assessment.[a] Typical questions in these domains may include:

F: Is faith (or spirituality) a part of your life, or was it in the past?[b] Were you raised in a particular faith tradition or religion, and are you practicing now? Do you consider yourself a spiritual person? What gives you hope, strength, and peace?

I: What importance does your faith or belief have in your life? How would you rate the importance of your faith or belief on a scale from zero to ten? Have your beliefs influenced how you are thinking about or dealing with your medical situation?

C: Are you part of a spiritual or religious community? Has it helped you with your current health issues, and how? Is there a group of people you really love or who are important to you? Are there people praying for you?

A: What role do your beliefs play in your healthcare decision-making? How would you like your healthcare team to use information about your spirituality and beliefs as we care for you?

LORD, developed by Dr. Walt Larimore, is an acronym for Lord, others, religious struggle, and do, and incorporates an assessment for spiritual distress. LORD questions may include:[c]

L: May I ask about your faith background? Do you have a spiritual or faith preference, now or in the past?

O: Do you meet with others in spiritual or religious community? If so, how often? How important is this to you?

R: Has this illness (or situation) caused you to question God's love for you? Do you feel that God (or Allah or a higher power) has abandoned you? Have you asked God to heal you and he hasn't? Do you believe God or the devil (or the spirit world) is punishing you for something?

D: What can I do to incorporate your faith (or spirituality) into your medical care? How might your beliefs influence our treatment decisions? Are there resources in your faith community you would like me to help mobilize for you? Would you like to see a chaplain (or pastor, priest, or imam) or religious counselor?

[a]Tami Borneman, Betty Ferrell, and Christina M. Pulchalski, "Evaluation of the FICA Tool for Spiritual Assessment," *Journal of Pain and Symptom Management* 40, no. 2 (2010): 163-73, http://doi.org/10.1016/j.jpainsymman.2009.12.019.
[b]I first heard the "Faith" question phrased this way by Dr. Shawn O'Driscoll.
[c]Walt Larimore, "Spiritual Assessment in Clinical Care, Part 2," *Today's Christian Doctor* (Fall 2015): 26-29, https://issuu.com/cmdacommunications/docs/tcd_fall_hi_res.

These standardized approaches include multiple sample questions, but typically I ask only one question for each letter in the acronym, and I often save some of the items for later in my patient interaction. It's helpful to choose the questions that work best for you in your context. If you learn from your initial question that your patient has never had an interest in spirituality, the subsequent questions typically become irrelevant. In this way the spiritual history is like other elements of a medical history: for instance, if a patient tells us they're not coughing, we don't ask follow-up questions about their sputum.

Here are a couple of spiritual histories I've taken recently, during the social history portion of an overall patient assessment:

Me: What kind of work have you done?
Patient: I'm a high school science teacher.
Me: Do you enjoy teaching?
Patient: Yes, very much so.
Me: Is faith a part of your life, or was it in the past?
Patient: I'm not into religion. When I was a kid my parents took me to church, but the people there were hypocrites.
Me: Thank you for sharing that with me. Tell me about your family. . . .

Me: Has faith been a part of your life?
Patient: Yes, I go to a Baptist church.
Me: How important is faith to you?
Patient: It's very important to me.

Me: Has your faith community been supportive of you recently?

Patient: Well, people say they're praying for me, but it doesn't seem to be helping.

Me: Wow, that's tough. Do you feel that God has abandoned you or is punishing you?

Patient: Sometimes.

Me: That must be difficult.

Patient: Yeah, it is.

Me: Thank you for sharing that with me. I'd like to ask about your family's medical history. . . .

The spiritual history gives us insight into the spirituality of our religious patients, but it can also give us a nuanced understanding of people with no religious affiliation, sometimes called "nones." They are a heterogeneous group with a wide range of perspectives on faith. Some are spiritual nihilists, convinced that there is no God or spiritual plane of reality. They hold that values and beliefs are ultimately baseless, that life is meaningless, and that science is the only reliable way to understand reality.[33] Although Christians often focus on how to engage with spiritual nihilists, they make up only 10 percent of American adults. Another group of nones are "spiritually curious." They are by far the largest group of nones in the United States, estimated to number one hundred million Americans.[34] They have in common an openness to and curiosity about spiritual reality. Some have roots in Christianity or another religion but have moved away from faith, and others have no religious background but are intrigued by spirituality. They have a range of worldviews and spiritual practices, and although they're attracted to spirituality, they may be wary of institutional religion. The spiritually curious are often less concerned with doctrine than with practical questions, such as, "Where can I find hope and meaning?" and, "What happens to me after I die?" They may be more interested in the journey than the destination, and they seek fellow travelers, not religious experts. They want to dialogue about faith, not listen to monologues.[35]

Your first spiritual history question—the *F* of FICA or the *L* of LORD— can be tailored to the patient population you serve. If you're working in a culture where most patients have a religious affiliation, and their religion is often apparent in the way they dress, the first question may more properly begin with a statement: "I see from your attire that you are Sikh. Is that right?" If, on the other hand, you're seeing millennial-generation patients in the context of a secular society, the question "Are you religious?" is likely to be answered "No," ending your spiritual history-taking without yielding nuanced insight into your patient's worldview. Questions such as "Has faith been a part of your life?" or "Do you have spiritual resources that help you in stressful times?" may yield a better understanding of your patient in some contexts.

Adapt the spiritual history to your particular work setting.[36] Here are some examples:

- A friend of mine who works in an emergency department says, "If the patient is here for suture removal or with a sprained ankle, the topic doesn't come up. But if they have a serious problem or their lifestyle led to their acute health issue, I'll ask 'Do you have any spiritual or faith practices?' as part of a social history—once the patient is stable."

- A colleague who manages chronic medical illness in an outpatient practice waits until a trusted relationship has developed, usually the patient's second or third clinic visit, to ask about spirituality. He often leads by saying, "Sometimes what's going on in our lives has an impact on the success of our treatment. What's going on in your life these days?" The response to this question sometimes reveals spiritual need.

- A nurse working in a pre-procedure area looks at his patient's intake questionnaire for their religious affiliation, and if they have an affiliation, asks whether their faith is important to them. Based on their response, he asks whether they would like prayer. He has now prayed with hundreds of patients.

- A physical therapist finds that some of her patients have a difficult time adjusting to the limitations they're facing. When she asks them, "Where do you look to for hope?" she gets various answers: "Friends and family." "I'm hoping I'll get back to normal." "I don't have any hope. It's hard." Some of her patients then ask her, "Where do you get hope from?" and she shares her own experience finding hope in God.

- After he's discussed his diagnostic impression and plan, another colleague says to his patients, "Now, let's talk about your soul."
- A coworker who transports patients around the hospital doesn't take a full spiritual history as he is pushing a patient's stretcher or wheelchair but does ask, "How is your spirit doing today?"

There are context-appropriate ways to assess patients' spiritual health, no matter what your healthcare role is.

Spiritual history dos and don'ts. The spiritual history is an assessment tool. It's not aimed at conversion. It consists of questions and does not include making statements beyond brief expressions of empathy. When taking a spiritual history you can say, "Tell me more about that," but you should avoid preaching, giving spiritual advice, or describing your own faith, religious practices, or theological views. Based on what you learn about a patient by taking their spiritual history, you may want to respond in a way that encourages their spiritual health. However, resist the temptation to jump to this immediately! Diagnosis precedes treatment. Take time to truly understand your patients' spiritual situation in the context of their overall health. Rather than responding right away, it may most benefit the patient to circle back to spiritual issues during a later part of your interaction with them—as we'll consider in subsequent chapters.

> When taking a spiritual history you can say, "Tell me more about that," but you should avoid preaching, giving spiritual advice, or describing your own faith, religious practices, or theological views.

We can explain why we're taking a spiritual history to patients who question its relevance or appropriateness, referring to the scientific evidence and best-practices guidelines we've already reviewed. We can also assure wary patients that they don't have to answer spiritual history questions. If you work in a healthcare organization that is suspicious of spirituality or concerned about staff attempting to convert patients to their own belief system, consider meeting with your supervisor, mentioning the relevant scientific evidence and guidelines, and explaining your interest in culturally competent patient care before you begin.

Time constraints. The spiritual history can seem like one more thing competing for inclusion in our hectic clinical days. We may feel that we simply don't have the time to take an interest in our patients' spiritual health. Yet caring for patients this way is an important source of fulfillment for us. How can we practice whole-person care efficiently?

The core of the spiritual history is one to four questions. Some patients will respond to our first question by indicating that they have no faith or current interest in spirituality: in this case you're done taking their spiritual history. Even in these cases, the mere fact that you've expressed an interest in your patient's spirituality may beneficially shape your relationship. Your patient has learned that you are interested in and value their whole person, which for some is an important factor in deciding to trust you—and trust is essential to productive and time-efficient patient relationships.

Taking a spiritual history usually takes less than thirty seconds. We learn some basic and relevant facts about the importance of faith in our patient's life and move on. When you first start taking spiritual histories the process may seem surprisingly simple and bland. It is nonetheless useful because it takes your patient's spiritual temperature, gives you opportunity to diagnose spiritual needs, and aligns you with God in the middle of your workflow.

> Taking a spiritual history usually takes less than thirty seconds. We learn some basic and relevant facts about the importance of faith in our patient's life and move on.

SOULS AND SPIRITS AT YOUR WORKPLACE

Much of the satisfaction we find in our work comes from the awareness we are caring for whole persons—bodies, souls, and spirits—even as we rightly focus on physical ailments. Here are some practical ways to develop your awareness of the souls and spirits of your patients:

Know that body, soul, and spirit issues often mingle. Our biology, psychology, and spirituality are tied together in each of us. They are inseparable aspects of our humanity. That's why illness can bring not only physical pain and suffering but also psychological and spiritual suffering that may include isolation, anxiety, and fear of separation and extinguishment. These different forms of suffering can amplify one another. A nursing colleague told me about a palliative care patient whose pain was not controlled by increasing doses of morphine. The nurse asked her whether she had a relationship that needed mending. "I haven't talked to my sister in years. How did you know?" the patient asked. "I can see that you are suffering," the nurse replied. She connected the patient to her sister by telephone and left the room. The patient's pain was well controlled thereafter.[37] We are better caregivers when we're alert to the possibility that psychological matters, social issues, or spiritual needs are affecting our patient's physical health.

Take pleasure in the immaterial dimensions of your work. Often it's the impact of our care on souls and spirits that most benefits our patients—even though it comes through treatment of a physical problem. A physician recently said to me, "I'm a human being working with other human beings, having relationships with them and helping them live happier lives. That's what brings me fulfillment." Recognize that satisfaction comes from a broader view of what you do, a view that requires a three-dimensional awareness of your patients. Incorporate assessments of psychological and spiritual health into your workflow, and celebrate the larger impact of your work.

Start taking your patients' spiritual temperature. This is a best practice in healthcare, and the evidence presented in this chapter supports including this in your clinical evaluations. In some cases you may sense spiritual need, distress, or interest, and taking a spiritual history becomes your means of further assessment. The spiritual history may seem especially appropriate when you are evaluating a new patient, when doing preventative healthcare assessments, when caring for a patient with a serious or chronic illness, or before major interventions. In some contexts a simpler approach—"How's your spirit doing?"—may suffice. But don't wait for an obvious indication to assess your patient's spirituality. Make it part of your routine.[38] You'll find that this practice gives you insight into your patients' lives, opens the door to encouraging their spiritual health in some cases, and reminds you of God's presence at work. Patient care takes on a new dimension as the spiritual plane of your work comes into view.

FOR REFLECTION

1. Describe what *soul* and *spirit* refer to.

2. Which elements of your workplace culture best affirm and nurture your own soul and spirit? Which elements need improvement?

3. Looking at the example of Elijah, how can body, soul, and spirit influence one another and a person's overall health? When have you seen one dimension of personhood impact the health of other dimensions?

4. Has your professional success exhausted you, like it did Elijah? To what extent is your fatigue due to bodily issues that we looked at in the last chapter, versus soul and spirit issues? If the weight of caregiving is draining you, consider jumping ahead to part three of this book.

5. What would you say to a patient or colleague who challenged your habit of taking a spiritual history?

IT'S YOUR TURN

For all of us, whether we're burned out or thriving in healthcare, our spirit mediates much of the satisfaction we draw from our careers. Don't let your spirit sleep through your workday. Rouse your spirit by exercising it:

1. Identify recurring moments during your day when you can pause for a few seconds to speak silently to God—perhaps when you're logging on to a computer, washing your hands, riding an elevator, waiting for a medication, or standing in line. Commit to touching base with God at least four times a day or shift. Tell him what's going on, ask him for what you need, and pause for a few seconds, giving him space to direct your thoughts. If you need help remembering,

use faith words in your medical record login password, or put "The LORD is the strength of my life" (Ps 27:1 KJV) on your phone lock screen and start your prayer with that phrase.

2. Your work affects the souls and spirits of patients and coworkers. Often it's how you do what you do that touches the spirits of others, and your own spirit can flourish as these beneficial interactions grow. When work seems routine or boring, try perceiving others as three-dimensional (body, soul, and spirit), not one-dimensional. Give people your full attention. Look at their eyes while they are speaking. Become a careful observer of others. Can you identify something distinctive about the soul and spirit of each of your patients?

3. Make spirituality a part of your routine workflow by taking spiritual histories. Like other skills, it takes practice. Remember, it's about asking questions, not expressing your own views! Try out various strategies listed in this chapter and learn which ones work best and feel most natural to you and your patients.

PART 2

Sickness and Health

4

Health and Healing

ONE MORNING, ON ROUNDS WITH MY TEAM, I met a homeless man who had been admitted to our service overnight with pneumonia. The intern mentioned that the patient had at one time had a job and an apartment, but he now slept under a highway overpass and panhandled on the sidewalk for money. We walked into his room and gathered around his bed. He looked up suspiciously at us, a company of white-coated professionals surrounding him. He was scrawny, with muscle wasting, suggesting malnutrition. He was also tremulous and anxious, and in addition to giving him antibiotics for pneumonia, we began treating him for alcohol withdrawal.

Over the following days he improved. His tremor resolved, his appetite came back, and he began to walk around the ward. A social worker and an alcohol use disorder counselor both came to see him, but he refused to work with them and signed out of the hospital against medical advice. My team and I failed to take a spiritual history, so I don't know whether he was open to spiritual resources that might have helped him. A few weeks later he was again admitted to our hospital, this time with major trauma after being hit by a motor vehicle.

Health is priceless. When we're healthy, our bodies, souls, and spirits are thriving. Health feels so natural, so right, that we tend to assume it's a permanent state of affairs—until we lose it. Treatment of a physical problem restores some of our patients to complete health, but others, like the patient I've described, continue to cope with ill health in other aspects of their lives, often with physical consequences. And when our own spirits are thwarted or dormant, we ourselves are not truly healthy, even though our biology may be functioning normally.

In a poll of American adults, over 90 percent of people agreed with the statement, "Health is so much more than just not being sick."[1] They said that health included things such as having a job, living independently, having friends, being calm, or being happy. The majority said they wished their healthcare professional would talk to them about social and integrative aspects of wellness. However, only 10 percent said that their caregiver asked what brings them happiness or joy, or discussed their spiritual health. Their healthcare professionals tended to focus on test results, medications, and exercise.[2]

These data show that our patients often have a broader view of health than we do, and that most of them would welcome conversations about spirituality. My daughter volunteers at a pregnancy support center. She says that many of the women who come for prenatal care have social, financial, and spiritual concerns. When she mentions that health has emotional and spiritual aspects, some of her clients talk about these concerns and how they affect their healthcare decisions. In this chapter we'll see that the biblical concepts of health and healing are broad, incorporating these elements and exemplifying ideas embraced by the World Health Organization.[3] We'll also look at practical ways to efficiently incorporate biblical approaches into our patient interactions. Thinking biblically about health can broaden our understanding of our purpose, make us better caregivers, and add a meaningful dimension to our careers.

THE BIBLICAL CONCEPTS OF HEALTH AND HEALING

The Bible uses a variety of words to describe health. The best known is the Hebrew word *shalom*, which can be translated as "well-being," "peace," "safety," "soundness," "prosperity," "intactness," "completeness," or "wholeness." Dr. Stan Haegert calls shalom "the sweet spot of life."[4] The biblical concept of health is broad, incorporating not only normal bodily functioning but also robust energy, freedom, peace, security, and prosperity. Job, reflecting on the wide range of human life experiences, describes people who enjoy these various aspects of health throughout life:

"One person dies in full vigor, completely secure and at ease, well nourished in body, bones rich with marrow" (Job 21:23-24). Jeremiah, prophesying during a time of war and captivity, quotes God's promise to restore and renew his people: "I will bring health and healing . . . ; I will heal my people and will let them enjoy abundant peace and security" (Jer 33:6). The Bible's Wisdom literature links body, soul, and spirit health (e.g., Prov 4:20-23; 17:22; see also 3 Jn 1:2). Right relationship with God brings health: "Do not be wise in your own eyes; fear the LORD and shun evil. This will be health to your body and nourishment to your bones" (Prov 3:7-8). Right social and societal relationships are also linked to health: "Blessed are those who have regard for the weak; the LORD delivers them in times of trouble. . . . The LORD sustains them on their sickbed and restores them from their bed of illness" (Ps 41:1, 3).

The healthy person has vigor and experiences peace, contentment, safety, and harmony with their environment, their community, and God. These various aspects of health are synergistic. Randomized controlled trials support this conclusion: spiritually based interventions decrease blood pressure in hypertensive patients, regular meditation is associated with improvements in blood sugar and hemoglobin A1C levels among diabetic patients, and spiritual and religious interventions decrease heart rate, anxiety, and depression in patients with cardiovascular diseases.[5] Robust social relationships are associated with improved physical health and longevity.[6] Perhaps you've noticed this synergy in your own health. I know that I'm more productive and sleep better when I'm exercising regularly and when I'm not in conflict with the people with whom I work, play, and worship. I also find that when I devote morning time to my relationship with God, I experience peace at critical moments of my workday. Health is a virtuous cycle involving body, soul, and spirit.

The biblical concept of healing is similarly broad. Consider, for example, these verses from the Psalms:

> The healthy person has vigor and experiences peace, contentment, safety, and harmony with their environment, their community, and God. These various aspects of health are synergistic.

Praise the LORD, my soul,
    and forget not all his benefits—
who forgives all your sins
    and heals all your diseases,
who redeems your life from the pit
    and crowns you with love and compassion,
who satisfies your desires with good things
    so that your youth is renewed like the eagle's. (Ps 103:2-5)

This passage describes benefits God gives his people, restoring them to shalom, including the resolution of disease but also much more: recovery of freedom and autonomy, experience of love and care, satisfaction of desires, and renewal of youth. It is God who forgives, heals, redeems, crowns, and satisfies us. "The pit" is a literal hole or cistern that people can't escape (see Gen 37:23-24); it's also a metaphor for any predicament we can't get ourselves out of (Job 9:31; 33:19-22; Ps 7:15; 28:1), including serious health issues. God is the one who secures our freedom and pulls us out of the pit. Human flourishing involves body, soul, and spirit. We are healthiest when all aspects of our personhood are thriving. We miss opportunities to heal whole persons when we mend patients' bodies but don't tend to turmoil affecting their souls or spirits.

BIOMEDICAL HEALING AND COMMON GRACE

It seems obvious that miraculous or supernatural healing, experienced in a church or by the intervention of a person with the spiritual gift of healing, comes from God. But what about the healing we routinely carry out in healthcare? Does God have anything to do with healing that comes via medicines, therapy, or surgery?

God is the source of all healing. He says, "I am the LORD, who heals you" (Ex 15:26). He is the one who "forgives all your sins and heals all your diseases" (Ps 103:3). Healing originates with God, regardless of whether it comes by miraculous or medical means.

> Healing originates with God, regardless of whether it comes by miraculous or medical means.

This is illustrated in the story of Hezekiah, a king of Israel who became seriously ill. Isaiah 38 dedicates twenty verses to the spiritual significance of his illness and God's role in his treatment, and only one verse to the medical facts of his case. When Hezekiah becomes sick, he repents, and God responds by saying, "I have heard your prayer and seen your tears; I will add fifteen years to your life" (Is 38:5). The chapter concludes with one sentence describing the medical aspect of his diagnosis and treatment: "Isaiah had said, 'Prepare a poultice of figs and apply it to the boil, and he will recover'" (Is 38:21). Fig extracts have antimicrobial properties, and it seems that application of a warm, hypertonic dressing to what may have been an abscess or cutaneous anthrax healed Hezekiah.[7] Yet after he is healed, Hezekiah says, "[God] himself has done this. . . . You restored me to health and let me live" (Is 38:15-16).

If I had been writing the account of Hezekiah's illness and its treatment, I might have devoted far more text to the medical details and less to his repentance and God's response! If I had been his caregiver, I might even have been blind to God's role in his healing, taking credit for his healing myself. God used human knowledge of medical technique to heal Hezekiah, and he uses healthcare to heal people today. The success of medications, therapy, and surgery in no way invalidates God's role in healing. "We treat, Jesus heals."[8]

Healing is part of God's common grace bestowed on humankind. The term "common grace" refers to God's beneficence toward all of his creation, including all people. The psalmist says that God "upholds *all* who fall" and "satisf[ies] the desires of *every* living thing" (Ps 145:14, 16, emphasis added). God demonstrates his love for all humanity through the ingenuity, skill, and insight he gifts people with, regardless of whether they believe in him.[9] For instance, the prophet Isaiah writes that God provides farmers with the technical knowledge and skills they need to produce bountiful crops (Is 28:24-29). Scientific knowledge and beneficial medical innovations are also gifts from God to all people. The God who "causes his sun to rise on the evil and the good" (Mt 5:45) is the one who has given humanity the insights and skills that make modern medical healing possible. "Every good and perfect gift is from above, coming down from the Father of the heavenly lights" (Jas 1:17). Among these gifts are our medical knowledge and our bodies' immunological and healing capacities, without which many of our treatments would fail. Medical healing is attributable to God. We healthcare professionals are instruments of his common grace.

WHOLE-PERSON HEALTHCARE
IN A BIOMEDICAL WORLD

The biblical concepts we've reviewed imply that physical healing is not an isolated end in itself. We work to improve our patients' bodily health so that they can enjoy life, live longer, be productive, realize their potential, find harmony with God and other people, and experience satisfaction through their own life and work. But a wounded soul or crippled spirit can hold our patients back. That's why times when we heal whole persons—affecting bodies, souls, and spirits for good—are memorable for healthcare workers. They fulfill our larger human purpose of restoring creation. They bring us joy.

We benefit when we approach our patients this way. However, our training and professional skillset are typically not designed to address the broader components of health. How can we begin to incorporate holistic approaches into our busy healthcare practices? We've already considered a few methods: calling out aspects of the image of God in our patients, or taking their spiritual history, or stating that health has emotional and spiritual aspects and asking how our patients are doing in these areas. The Bible offers us additional strategies.

> Times when we heal whole persons—affecting bodies, souls, and spirits for good—are memorable for healthcare workers. They fulfill our larger human purpose of restoring creation. They bring us joy.

Speaking gracious words. Proverbs tell us that the way we speak to our patients can contribute to healing:

> The words of the reckless pierce like swords,
>   but the tongue of the wise brings healing. (Prov 12:18)

> Gracious words are a honeycomb,
>   sweet to the soul and healing to the bones. (Prov 16:24)

Our bedside manner has the power to heal or to harm. Healing comes through medicines and surgery, and also through our words and non-verbal communication. Gracious words can reveal Jesus' love to our patients, particularly when our words cut across a current of prejudice, guilt, discouragement, or shame. They bring encouragement and hope. They are "sweet to the soul." These words often come from our own careful observation: when we notice glimmers of patience, honesty, graciousness, or strength in our patients, we can tell them about it.

We have many opportunities to speak wisely in clinical settings. We speak wise words when we take our patients' concerns seriously, and chart a path that addresses them. As we learn about their most important relationships and observe their interactions with family and friends, we can reflect back to our patients their importance in the lives of other people. When appropriate, we can encourage our patients that they will recover, that their symptoms will improve or that their strength will return, and that they can make a fresh start. Sometimes wise words draw attention to emotional and spiritual pathways to health.

Giving God credit for healing. We have this opportunity when our patients thank us for our care. After all, God provided the knowledge, skills, and intrinsic biological healing mechanisms that enable us to care for our patients successfully. After graciously accepting our patients' thanks, we can direct it beyond ourselves. One colleague of mine starts by acknowledging her coworkers: "I feel so blessed to be part of your care team." She then goes on to reflect gratitude toward God, saying, "I thank God things have gone so well for you," or "I think God has done something special for you." Another colleague tells his patients, "Someone upstairs has been looking out for you." When we start to feel wise in our own eyes, congratulating ourselves for successful patient outcomes but not giving God credit, our own soul health and spirit health are in jeopardy. In the long run, satisfaction best comes from knowing that God is at work through us.

Offering faith perspectives. The Bible gives counsel about many issues our patients (or their families) commonly struggle with. When we hear about these, we can offer biblical perspectives, with the goal of enhancing our patients' spiritual wellbeing. Even in a rapid-fire work environment,

God may prompt you to take a minute with occasional patients to gently supplement the understanding of someone who is:

- experiencing regret
- feeling their worth is diminished by their illness
- believing God has abandoned them or is punishing them with illness
- wondering whether there is a God powerful enough to undo the evil that is afflicting them
- wanting to reconnect with God after neglecting their spirituality for years but feeling they are unworthy
- wondering how they will deal with the financial consequences of illness and its treatment
- questioning how God can allow suffering
- thinking they must choose between prayer and medicine
- sensing their own spirituality while out in nature or listening to music and now wanting to know more
- seeing no path to forgiveness and reconciliation in their most important relationships
- sensing there must be something more to life

Sometimes we discover that our patients are struggling with issues such as these by asking, "How are you processing this situation?" or "What's on your mind these days?" Our best initial response is often simply to empathize, responding by saying, "That must be hard," "That's a difficult place to be," or "You're dealing with some tough issues." If we're in the middle of evaluating the patient or performing a healthcare task, we might then move on, circling back to the matter later—for instance, when we're discussing their diagnosis or treatment. At that point, spiritual concerns can join physical matters on our problem list.

We can handle our patients' spiritual needs in several ways. Asking follow-up questions is often helpful, because questions can reveal the complexity of the patient's concerns. Once we appreciate their situation, we might choose to offer forward-looking encouragement and guidance from our own perspective. We might say something like, "Your concerns are real, and I don't know how they will all work out. But I do think there is a God who cares about you and will provide for you one day at a time," or "A verse from my own faith background that's been useful to me in difficult times is . . . ," or "You're dealing with some important spiritual issues. Have you ever felt God speaking to you about things like this, now or in the past?" Another option is to refer the patient to a chaplain, religious professional, or counselor for help, much as we would refer patients to consultants for help with problems that lie outside our own expertise or scope of practice. This may be our best option when we're pressed for time or don't feel we can address the patient's issue. You'll begin to make these referrals once you start consistently taking spiritual histories, and it's good to talk to relevant professionals (such as your hospital chaplains or a visitation pastor) ahead of time to best understand what they can offer and how to refer patients to them.

For patients from a faith tradition different from your own, be prepared to offer referral to a counselor or spiritual professional from their own faith. This is particularly important if you work in a secular context. In these settings, our role is typically to encourage and model healthy spirituality and to invite questions about spirituality—not to persuade our patients to convert to our own religion. God often uses a number of people and circumstances to bring individuals to himself over time, and while we aim to be part of that process, the final outcome is not up to us. When we offer the option of a referral within our patient's own faith tradition, we verbalize what they may already be thinking, we find out whether they're comfortable with their own faith community or alienated from it, and we demonstrate respect and care for them even as we affirm the importance of spirituality. Rather than closing a door, we're creating an avenue for future interaction. After referring patients, we can follow up with them about their spiritual issues just as we would follow up about other diagnoses.

Encouraging spiritual health. Some of our patients are contemplating a future that looks different than they had imagined. They may be realizing for the first time that they're not in control of their own destiny or that life will not be all they had planned for. Some respond fatalistically or bitterly to these disappointments. Others opt for passivity, feeling like putty in the hands of their healthcare professionals. Yet the healthiest response, the response that will best serve our patients, is to look forward with a sense of gratitude and hope. They can certainly hope in the effectiveness of medical treatments, and we will leverage these for maximum benefit. They need also to take renewed ownership of their spirituality. A healthy spirit best equips them to navigate the future, seeing what is possible and not missing what a loving God has in store.

The practice of gratitude is both a religious and secular window into spirituality, and encouraging gratitude is one method of influencing our patients' outlook. Paul, under house arrest and contemplating the possibility of being sentenced to death, writes, "Do not be anxious about anything, but in every situation, by prayer and petition, *with thanksgiving*, present your requests to God. And the peace of God, which transcends all understanding, will guard your hearts and your minds in Christ Jesus" (Phil 4:6-7, emphasis added). He knew from personal experience that thankfulness in prayer was an important pathway to peace in the face of adversity. Similarly, biomedical research has linked gratitude to changes in brain function, improved healthcare outcomes, and decreased mortality in healthy populations over time.[10] To our patients, it may seem paradoxical or even absurd to suggest that they express gratitude, but science shows that this practice can result in improved physical and psychological health. We can suggest practical strategies, such as regularly expressing thankfulness to God in prayer, writing a weekly gratitude letter to another person, or keeping a gratitude journal—in any of these ways, finding things in each day to appreciate and be thankful for.[11]

Research also shows that nurses who habitually express gratitude perform better in high-pressure clinical situations.[12] For both us and our patients, the expression of gratitude can shift our frame of mind, remind us of the beauty of daily life, renew our connection to our Creator, and bring us peace and clarity in difficult times.

We rightly focus on our patients' specific medical problems. After all, that is why they're seeing us. But when we also consider their soul and spirit, we remind ourselves of biblical concepts of health and healing and align ourselves with God in real time. When we aim to heal whole persons—using simple strategies that encourage our patients' spirits—we best fulfill our purpose and find satisfaction.

FOR REFLECTION

1. Are you healthy yourself? Remember that health incorporates physical, emotional, psychological, nutritional, material, social, and spiritual components. If you are healthy, you are in harmony with other people and God. How are you doing in each of these areas? What's needed for you to thrive in this way?

2. Gracious words, giving God credit for healing, offering biblical perspectives, and encouraging gratitude can all bring healing to our patients. Which of these do you practice already? How can you implement additional elements into your practice in time-efficient and context-appropriate ways? Review the examples mentioned in the latter half of this chapter. Could these be a source of satisfaction in your healthcare career?

IT'S YOUR TURN

We are not fully comfortable with new healthcare methods until we've used them at work. It's the same with the ideas in this book: we have to put them into practice to discover the difference they can make. Pick one or more of the following activities and make them a daily habit this week:

1. Take the initiative to improve one aspect of your own soul health and spirit health. This might involve starting each day by praying and meditating on a passage of Scripture, singing or listening to worship songs during your commute, looking to God when you're in the middle of a difficult situation, talking to someone you trust about a feeling you're struggling with, investing time and attention in an important relationship, apologizing to someone you've hurt, or practicing gratitude.

2. Your work can be an important contributor to your overall satisfaction in life. But it is God—not our work primarily—who satisfies our desires with good things (Ps 103:5). This week, tell God about

your work-related longings and desires, and ask him to shape them and fulfill them.

3. Speak wise words to your patients that draw attention to the image of God within them. Reflect back to them their bravery, patience, gentleness, or strength. Compliment their humor, stamina, or forbearance. Ask them how their spirit is doing. In these moments, your spirit is speaking to their spirit. This simple practice reminds us that we are more than technical experts. We are human beings healing fellow humans.

4. Give God credit for the healing your patients experience. Find appropriate ways to express this in response to your patients' thanks, starting with the examples given in this chapter.

5. When you think it would be helpful, encourage your patients to practice gratitude. One way to raise this subject is to ask, "Is there anything you're grateful for today?" Be ready to explain that science links gratitude to improved health outcomes and that spiritual and physical health are intertwined. Depending on their spiritual history, consider recommending a gratitude journal, gratitude letters, or regularly giving thanks in prayer.

5

"Why Me?"

As an intern I cared for a young woman with acute leukemia who was hospitalized with fever. She had been diagnosed during her sophomore year of college and had entered remission after her initial course of chemotherapy, but the leukemia had quickly relapsed. She was now receiving a second-line treatment regimen that had suppressed her white blood cell count, and she was vulnerable to infection. Although she was pale, her cheeks were flushed, and she was febrile, tachycardic, and weak. I sent cultures and started her on intravenous fluids and antibiotics.

In the hospital she kept a Bible on her bedside table. I learned that she loved music and sang in her church choir. Her church community was the core of her social circle, and she frequently had visitors, including her family and friends. However, these visits did not seem to be happy events for my patient. When I entered her room during visiting hours I encountered silence, not conversation. Her visitors sat glumly by her bedside, and she would be looking out the window.

One afternoon I found my patient alone in her room, her cheeks wet with tears. I asked her why she was crying. "My family says God would heal me if I would only confess all the sin in my life," she said. "The problem is, I can't think of any more sin to confess."

How would you respond to my patient? Her dilemma exposes questions that she and many others ask themselves: Why did I get sick? How can I be healed? She had already heard medical answers about the cause of her disease and the effectiveness of treatments, but she was struggling

with the significance of her illness at a spiritual level. Some of our patients—including some who are without religious affiliation but spiritually curious—are asking themselves similar questions about the
meaning of their illness and the lack of hope they feel.

It can be daunting to imagine responding to our patients' "Why me?"
In this chapter we'll look at biblical answers to this question and how they
equip us to simply and effectively encourage our patients' spiritual health.
Recognizing a patient's spiritual turmoil, and responding helpfully instead of sidestepping their concerns, can amplify the fulfillment we get
from healthcare work.

THE HOW AND THE WHY

Medicine and Scripture both give powerful insights into illness. Their approaches to disease are complementary. Biomedical science reveals *how*
illness occurs. The Bible displays a nuanced understanding of the how of
sickness, recognizing physical and psychological causes (Mt 4:24), but
also offers insight into the meaning and spiritual significance of sickness—
the *why* of human suffering. The biblical account of illness portrays how
sickness entered the human experience (the curse), considers the link
between our behavior and some individual illnesses (our shortcomings),
and offers forward-looking answers about the meaning of sickness (God
at work). We'll look at these in turn. They each speak to issues some of
our patients contend with. It turns out that a correct spiritual understanding of sickness is an important source of hope in healthcare settings,
for our patients and for us.

THE CURSE

We all commonly care for patients who are sick through no fault of their
own. We can trace the origin of these illnesses back to the curses placed
on all of creation in the early chapters of the Bible. According to Genesis,
pain, suffering, and death entered the human experience through the actions of Adam and Eve. They lived in a paradise, and they were in harmony
with their ecosystem, God, and each other until they chose to disobey
God. Their actions brought shame on them and broke their relationship

with God, who expelled them from the Garden of Eden. Their resulting separation from the immediate presence and experience of God had a cascading impact on their lives, summarized in the curses of Genesis 3. They now had a broken relationship not only with God but also with the creation they were meant to tend and enjoy, which produced thorns and thistles. Their human relationships were broken, culminating in their son Cain's murder of his brother. Their self-understanding was marred by guilt and shame, and their experience of health was interrupted by pain, not only in illness and childbearing but also in the course of their daily work.[1] The final result of the curse was death.

All human suffering can be traced back to the brokenness and separation Genesis describes, brokenness that is inevitably recapitulated in our own experiences (Rom 5:14; 8:10). We are programmed to age and subject to death. The curse's effects seem particularly obvious in inherited diseases, diseases of childhood, or illnesses and trauma that result from the harmful actions of others, but the curse is the spiritual root of all the illnesses we treat.

In most cases, our patients' suffering is the result of forces beyond their control and is not tied to their own decisions or behavior. Illness and death are part of the human experience because we live in a broken world (Rom 5:12). All creation groans under that burden, and we groan too, suffering under its weight (Rom 8:22-23). Even when our bodies are healthy, many of us are under the sway of the subconscious fear of death, meaning that the reality of death influences our outlook and drives our actions (more about that in chapter seven).

OUR SHORTCOMINGS

We also care for patients whose illnesses are linked to their own behaviors. For instance, patients who smoke, drive while inebriated, are sexually promiscuous, or ignore medical advice may suffer sickness or trauma as a result. Similarly, the Bible draws a cause-and-effect link between our choices and some illnesses. It calls these shortcomings *sin*.

Although the word *sin* may seem antiquated, the concept is alive and well today. The Hebrew word translated "sin" refers to missing the mark. It can refer to missing a target with a slingshot (Judg 20:16) or losing one's way in life out of ignorance and hastiness (Prov 19:2).[2] In my attitudes, words, and actions, I've often missed the mark by failing to think and do what's best. Even in postmodern cultures, most people have moral and ethical standards: they draw the line between acceptable and unacceptable behavior somewhere. Most will also admit that they've sometimes fallen short of their own standards. And, they recognize that poor choices may have adverse consequences. Many think that they will one day be judged for their shortcomings.[3]

The Pentateuch tells of times when God sent plagues and envenomations on Israelites who spoke against him or worshiped idols (Ex 32:35; Num 21:6). In the Old Testament there are accounts of God inflicting illness on rulers because of their misdeeds, which typically included leading their nation away from God. For instance, Jehoram was a king of Judah who murdered his brothers and encouraged idol worship. Elijah prophesied that he would be afflicted with a "lingering disease of the bowels" because of his immorality (2 Chron 21:15). The disease did occur, and after two years of illness Jehoram's "bowels came out . . . and he died in great pain" (2 Chron 21:19). Scripture relates instances of cardiovascular, gastrointestinal, dermatologic, toxic, and ophthalmologic afflictions linked to individual or community-wide sin. Sometimes it recognizes a biological mechanism (such as snakebite or tainted water) by which these afflictions occur. We shouldn't think that just a few diseases with an obvious pathophysiologic link to personal behavior (such as lung disease related to smoking) might be related to our own shortcomings.

A direct link between personal shortcomings and illness or death is also described in the New Testament (e.g., Acts 5:1-11). Paul writes about people who became sick or died because they took Communion as though it were a private party without recognizing its spiritual and communal significance (1 Cor 11:17-32). They were harming rather than building up the church. By disrespecting the sacrament of Communion, they chose "to share in the guilt of those responsible for the crucifixion, rather than by faith to receive the benefits of Jesus's sacrifice."[4]

It's important to understand that in this instance, sickness is not portrayed as condemnation by God. Paul characterizes these afflictions as the natural consequence of people's own actions. He then describes them as correction that will save people from ultimate condemnation: "When we are judged in this way by the Lord, we are being disciplined so that we will not be finally condemned with the world" (1 Cor 11:32). For Christ-followers there is no condemnation by God for sin (Rom 8:1-2), and nothing can separate us from the love of God (Rom 8:8-39). Far from being condemnation, sickness in this case is itself part of a remedy. It is a wakeup call that hopefully gets our attention and prompts change. Much as a wise parent disciplines their child for the child's own good, God's discipline is a result of his love for us (Rev 3:19).

Just as a bout of pneumonia may motivate a smoker to quit smoking, or the pain of a pulled muscle may lead us to regularly stretch and strengthen our muscles thereafter, a brush with mortality can prompt our patients to renew their relationship with God. This was true for a colleague of mine, who unexpectedly fell ill while at a medical conference on another continent. Alone in his hospital bed in a foreign country, far from his family and receiving treatments he was unfamiliar with, he realized how contingent his life was. He consulted me about his illness shortly after he returned home. He quickly returned to bodily health, but we both realized how shaken he felt. I invited him to join a Bible discussion group my wife and I were organizing. He accepted our invitation and actively participated in our group. Recentering his life around faith in Jesus released him from the looming fear of death he had acquired.

> A brush with mortality can prompt our patients to renew their relationship with God.

GOD AT WORK

Sickness is sometimes a sign that God is at work. In one well-known example, the Gospel of John relates the case of a man with congenital blindness who met Jesus:

> As he went along, [Jesus] saw a man blind from birth. His disciples asked him, "Rabbi, who sinned, this man or his parents, that he was born blind?"
>
> "Neither this man nor his parents sinned," said Jesus, "but this happened so that the works of God might be displayed in him. As long as it is day, we

must do the works of him who sent me. Night is coming, when no one can work. While I am in the world, I am the light of the world."

After saying this, he spit on the ground, made some mud with the saliva, and put it on the man's eyes. "Go," he told him, "wash in the Pool of Siloam" (this word means "Sent"). So the man went and washed, and came home seeing. (Jn 9:1-7)

The disciples seem to have thought that all health issues were linked to personal sin. In this case of congenital disability, they debated whether the man had somehow sinned while in utero or whether his disability was attributable to his parents' sins.[5] Jesus broadens their thinking. He says that the man's blindness was not due to his or his parents' sin but happened "so that the works of God might be displayed in him." Although all illness is an indirect consequence of Adam and Eve's original disobedience, Jesus here teaches us that disability may not be linked to individual shortcomings but is instead an opportunity for the work of God to be displayed through the life of the affected person. This man's miraculous healing displayed the power, grace, and true identity of Jesus to the disciples and the religious authorities of his day, as described in the rest of the passage.

The spiritual significance of illness may be to display God at work, even when healing doesn't occur. This was Paul's personal experience. He writes:

In order to keep me from becoming conceited, I was given a thorn in my flesh, a messenger of Satan, to torment me. Three times I pleaded with the Lord to take it away from me. But he said to me, "My grace is sufficient for you, for my power is made perfect in weakness." Therefore I will boast all the more gladly about my weaknesses, so that Christ's power may rest on me. That is why, for Christ's sake, I delight in weaknesses, in insults, in hardships, in persecutions, in difficulties. For when I am weak, then I am strong. (2 Cor 12:7-10)

While there is debate about the meaning of "thorn in the flesh," it's likely that Paul's affliction was physical and chronic. It tormented him. In response to his prayers, God told him that he was not going to heal him because there was a divine purpose for his affliction. Paul found that through his disability the power of God was displayed in his work and life (1 Cor 1:17; Gal 4:13-15). Joni Eareckson Tada is a similar, modern example.[6] At age seventeen she became quadriplegic due to a C4 spinal-cord injury caused by a diving accident. She prayed for physical healing but did not receive it. Since then, through books, artwork, and film, she has encouraged people who are struggling with disability and depression. She is an effective public advocate for people with disabilities, and her ministry Joni and Friends has brought physical aid, hope, and faith to thousands of people all over the world.

Jesus' comment that the blind man's disability "happened so that the works of God might be displayed in him" encourages us to look ahead for the spiritual purpose of our patients' afflictions rather than looking back in time for the factors that led to the condition. C. S. Lewis comments, "The disciples were not told *why* (in terms of efficient cause) the man was born blind: only the final cause, that the works of God be made manifest in him."[7] When it comes to the biology of illness, we search out the mechanism that led to our patient's sickness—the "efficient cause"—in order to understand and best treat it; but when it comes to the meaning of illness, Jesus refutes our tendency to look to the past and encourages us to look forward instead.[8] This is an important basis for hope in health-care settings, for our patients and for us.

> When it comes to the meaning of illness, Jesus refutes our tendency to look to the past and encourages us to look forward instead.

SHOULD WE ATTRIBUTE AN ILLNESS TO A SPECIFIC SPIRITUAL CAUSE?

Broadly speaking, the Bible gives us three strains of the meaning of sickness: the curse, our shortcomings, and God at work. It's tempting to assign one of these meanings to individual patients based on what we know about their personal histories and disease processes. But we can easily be wrong when we decide that one of these themes is dominant in a particular person's illness. Take, for example, Job's friends, who spend much of the book of Job wrongly counseling him that he has brought his illness on himself, or the disciples in John 9, who were sure the man's blindness was the result of individual sin. Getting this wrong can lead us to unconsciously judge our patients or misunderstand their needs. We can't be sure to what extent each of these three elements of spiritual pathophysiology is at play in the lives of an individual patient. God's ways are beyond our understanding (Is 55:8-9; Rom 11:33-36). It's best to avoid jumping to conclusions about the spiritual significance of our patients' illnesses.

What's more, these three biblical narratives about sickness are not mutually exclusive. All three may appear in the plot of an illness. We can always trace our patients' afflictions to the curse, which is the root of all human pain and suffering. Any illness might also be a wakeup call from God, an occurrence that prompts spiritual renewal. Furthermore, any illness might also be a venue for displaying the work of God. In fact, the narrative sweep of the entire Bible is about God repairing the brokenness of our world—a project that we, as healthcare workers, participate in daily. God's mercy is the overriding factor that allows us and our patients to respond to illness with hope.

WHY CARE ABOUT "WHY ME?"

Our workdays are full of the physical needs of our patients. For some of them, "Why me?" is not on their mind, and the topic doesn't come up. And for me, running behind schedule in clinic, it's easy to overlook the hints some patients drop that they are in spiritual turmoil. But when I do notice that a patient is troubled by "Why me?" and help them make progress, I experience the fulfillment that follows from aligning with God in the middle of my workflow. Noticing and responding to a patient's "Why me?" fulfills my broader purpose and brings me satisfaction.

Here are practical means of applying this chapter's concepts to our healthcare practices:

Be ready to respond to "Why me?" If you're taking spiritual histories and showing empathy to patients struggling with spiritual issues, some of them will ask you, "Why me?" When you hear this question from your patients, it's a sign that you are practicing spiritual care.[9] You might be tempted to respond with a biological explanation or a theology lesson, but when you recognize your patient is asking a spiritual question, you might choose to simply say, "I don't know." This is an honest response: we can't be sure of the relative roles of the curse, our shortcomings, and God at work in the situation of any individual patient. But we don't have to stop with "I don't know." We have an opportunity to help our patient move past their spiritual distress.

There are several ways to continue. You might ask, "What do you think about that?" The patient's answer may give you insight into their spiritual condition or reveal misperceptions. You could also circle back to the spiritual history. If they believe in God, as most people do, you might say, "I don't know why this has happened to you. But I do think that God loves you and is close to you." You might share your own experience: "I don't know why you're sick. But I know I wouldn't have made it through difficult times in my own life without knowing that God was near and that he cared." Dr. Harvey Elder's response to "Why me?" may be appropriate for some of your patients: "You were made for heaven, but you're stuck here on earth."[10] If the conversation progresses, you might offer a referral: "I sense that you're struggling with some important emotional and spiritual issues. Can we make a plan to address those with the help of a pastor or counselor?" If you are working in a culture that casts spiritual issues in terms of power and fear, you might say, "I don't know why this has happened to you. But I do know that God is more powerful than the forces of evil, that he cares about you, and that he is ready to walk with you through this illness."

Some of our patients have already settled on the why of their illness. The Bible may offer them a truer, more hopeful story. Common misconstruals of the meaning of sickness arise from spiritual distress, spiritual nihilism, and moral legalism.

Respond to spiritual distress. Spiritual distress, also called religious struggle, arises from the belief that illness signals God's abandonment or condemnation, or is a sign that God no longer loves the sick person or that demons or Satan are responsible for the illness. The young woman with leukemia I described at the start of this chapter was suffering from spiritual distress. This condition can affect persons from various religious traditions, as well as people without religious affiliation who are spiritually curious. In chapter three we considered how to ask patients about spiritual distress and reviewed the evidence that it is negatively associated with important health outcomes.

Our response to such patients will vary based on what we've learned by taking their spiritual history. Often our best first responses are empathic comments and more questions, aimed at coming to a better understanding of their situation. We can ask about spiritual resources in their life and offer referral to a religious counselor. We can choose to ask, "Would you like to know what I think about that?" and, with their permission, affirm that God has not abandoned them—he is close to them and continues to love them. To a Muslim woman who felt judged and abandoned by God and her faith community because of her illness, a surgeon I know asked, "Have you heard of Hagar?" He then went on to tell her the story of Hagar found in Genesis 16. She was abandoned by her community, including Abraham (the father of her son), and was alone with her child in the wilderness—but God had not forgotten her. He comforted her, restored her to her community, and turned her descendants into a great nation. To the young woman with leukemia whom I described at the start of this chapter, I said, "It must be very difficult to feel that way. I am sure that you are trying your best. Are you starting to wonder if God hears your prayers?" After listening to more of her story, I offered to pray with her, and I asked whether she would like my own pastor to visit her.

Respond to spiritual nihilism. In contrast to spiritual distress, which is a misperception of spiritual reality, spiritual nihilism is the belief that there is no spiritual reality. While most people believe in the existence of a deity, nihilists maintain that the physical universe is all there is: God doesn't exist, and human beings don't have spirits. A corollary of this belief is that there is no ultimate purpose to life. For spiritual nihilists, sickness doesn't have significance. It is meaningless, like all of human existence.

One convert to spiritual nihilism writes, "In the past I was constantly worried. I would berate myself for not being good enough. . . . Then, I found nihilism, and it was like a weight lifted off of my shoulders. No matter what life throws at me, I have the ultimate weapon: indifference."[11] Indifference may seem preferable to guilt and shame, and may in fact be a helpful response to some of life's

> Nihilism can leave our patients without the motivation to participate in their own care and without the perseverance that hope inspires.

difficulties, but it is an inadequate response to serious or chronic illness. Nihilism can leave our patients without the motivation to participate in their own care and without the perseverance that hope inspires.

Philosophical responses to spiritual nihilism include the argument from design, which posits that the existence, structure, and operation of both the universe and the human body are best explained by the existence of an intelligent designer. However, when caring for patients who are spiritual nihilists, our best response is usually not philosophical argument but rather affirmation of the reality of the nonmaterial aspects of existence. The experience of beauty, for instance, is an intangible but real phenomenon. We derive pleasure and satisfaction from beautiful things. When we put beautiful art in our clinic space, bring someone flowers, or play uplifting music, we affirm that beauty has meaning.[12] Compassion is also intangible but real, and when we treat our patients lovingly they may experience the reality of one spirit caring for another. Another way to point to spiritual reality is to notice and affirm aspects of the image of God in our patients, awakening in them the insight that they are more than biological machines.

These sorts of interactions can be fulcrums that pivot the perspective of spiritual nihilists. When they experience what Os Guinness calls "signals of transcendence," which are moments that point to the existence of good, evil, beauty, or love, they may stop being skeptical of spirituality and instead become seekers of meaning. Illness may itself be a signal that prompts our nihilist patients to acknowledge their need for significance. Christianity in particular offers nihilists an understanding of the world that explains both its brokenness and its beauty.[13]

Depending on your work context and your relationship with the patient, you might consider telling a spiritual nihilist that you pray for your patients and asking whether it would be OK if you put them on your prayer list. Or there may be times when it's appropriate to say, "I've noticed that some of my patients start asking themselves questions about the meaning of life at times like this. If that's happening and you'd like some help processing it, let me know." Raise these ideas in such a way that the patient can decline your offer without feeling that they have jeopardized their relationship with you or lost your interest. These expressions, particularly when made in the context of a trusted relationship and combined with demonstrations of goodness and compassion, may affect our patients for good.[14]

Anticipate moral legalism. Many people believe that the problems we experience are repayment for our previous misdeeds. They assume that our shortcomings result in an IOU that comes due, sooner or later, as personal misfortune or disaster. This is a common expression of human moral intuition, even among people without religious affiliation: 45 percent of all American adults believe that they will be judged for their decisions made here on earth.[15] A podcaster, speaking about women's attitudes toward bearing children in modern-day China, relates, "Even now, if you don't have a boy, you must have done something wrong in your previous life or your current life."[16] The belief that moral bookkeeping explains our disappointments drains people's hope—the past can't be changed, and it has determined our future—and contributes to their suffering.

There is, of course, a mechanistic link between some behaviors and illness. For instance, unhealthy diets and chronic tobacco or alcohol use are associated with a variety of health consequences. Yet our patients may understand their unhealthy behavior not as a risk factor contributing to the complex development of a disease but as the all-determining cause. Even in the absence of a plausible biologic link between their behavior and their illness, many patients believe their illness is payback for their shortcomings, a sort of cosmic retribution. The Bible does describe the moral debt that our actions incur and the real-world consequences we suffer, but it offers a fuller understanding. Morally speaking, the Bible teaches that we're all hopelessly in the red—but we all benefit from God's unmerited favor (Ps 130:3-4; 145:14; Lk 13:6-9). We don't deserve God's patience, compassion, and forgiveness, but he offers them to us anyway. He is reconciling the world to himself, "not counting people's sins against them" (2 Cor 5:19). Moral legalism misses God's mercy, forgiveness, and redemptive power.

To assess whether our patients are suffering from moral legalism, we might ask, "Why do you think this happened to you?" but the question may be awkward when there is an obvious behavioral risk factor (such as chronic medical noncompliance or substance use) that predisposed to their condition. I tend to assume that many of my patients view their situation through a lens of moral legalism and to respond proactively with grace and a forward outlook.

When I think it's true, I will sometimes tell a patient, "I don't think you did anything to cause this illness." A look of relief may cross their face. Occasionally I get a quizzical look or a question, in which case I'll explain that I know many of my patients worry about that. Sometimes a story of spiritual distress emerges. Occasionally I'll be asked, "Why me, then?" We earlier considered possible answers.

Choose grace. People who suffer from illness that is tied to their own choices and behavior often struggle with shame and regret. In addition, their healthcare professionals may have implicit biases against them—for instance, when illness is associated with substance use, risky behaviors, an unhealthy diet, or inattention to medical care.

If God is loving our patients, not condemning them, we can choose to love them too. Because we've experienced God's unmerited favor in our own lives, Christians have a special capacity to show favor to such patients. We do so by treating them with respect, getting to know them, perceiving elements of the image of God in them, and demonstrating acceptance and love in our manner and personal approach. When we treat them warmly, we gain: we experience the satisfaction that comes from being conduits of God's grace.

Our patients may respond by talking about their regrets. When that happens I sometimes reply, "We've all done things in our past we would now do differently. I certainly have." Depending on what I've learned from taking their spiritual history, I may add, "Fortunately, God is all about second chances."

Encourage patients to look forward, not backward. We can be confident that God is working out his intentions in our patients' lives. This doesn't mean that we should rush to assure them that God will heal them. We know that he may not. Reassurances such as "It will all work out," or "I'm sure you'll do fine," or "God works everything together for good," are not helpful when offered glibly or as shortcuts to the end of an uncomfortable conversation. Although we may not know what God's specific purpose is, we can be sure he wants our patients to draw close to him and to experience his peace. Often the first practical step is to encourage our patients to look beyond their current situation, with hope, both because of medical treatment and because God loves, forgives, and renews. We can get at what God is doing in their lives by asking, "Is this illness changing your priorities?" or "Is it affecting your approach to life [or work, or business, or family]?" or "Have you had a chance to connect with your spiritual side lately?"

By taking an interest in whole persons, we get glimpses of what God is doing through the illness we're treating. We are agents of grace, on the lookout for God's fingerprints. For instance, I learned that one of my patients worked in the sort of international, resource-limited settings where I've worked. After reading a book I mentioned, he made changes to his work that reflected a biblical approach and increased its beneficial impact in the lives of poor people. His chronic illness was never cured, but he blessed many people. I had the pleasure of encouraging him simply by reflecting back to him how God was using him to touch many other lives.

Affirm that, regardless of the why, God is close to our patients. The spiritual story of illness is a narrative of God at work in the lives of our patients—whether or not they believe in him. God is near to those who are suffering (Ps 10:14; 34:18). Far from abandoning them to illness, God is close to our patients. He is at work in our wards, clinics, consultation rooms, emergency departments, operating rooms, and home visits. He wants our patients to turn to him. Rather than dwelling on the role of a patient's past choices in their current situation, we can develop the habits of recognizing God's presence, looking for opportunities to assure our patients that God is near, and encouraging them to look ahead and look to him. A chemotherapy nurse I know tells patients who are in spiritual distress, "I don't think God has abandoned you or that your cancer is a punishment. I think God has brought you here because he has a purpose for you going forward." When they ask what that purpose is, she says, "Let's both pray that he will show it to you."

FOR REFLECTION

1. Do you think that illness occurs by chance? Do you think that every illness has a purpose? Could these both be true?

2. To what extent might we seek to determine whether the meaning of sickness is directly linked to personal shortcomings? Can we really know in any specific circumstance?

3. How do we best treat patients whose illnesses are medically linked to their own poor choices? Should we treat them differently from other patients? Could responding to these patients become a source of satisfaction (rather than frustration) for you?

4. If a patient told you that God had abandoned them or was punishing them, how would you respond?

IT'S YOUR TURN

Grace is unmerited favor, shown to others. Showing grace to others is key to your own spiritual health (Mt 18:21-35, the parable of the unmerciful servant). Find opportunities to put grace into practice with your patients:

1. Discover the issues your patients commonly cope with regarding the "why" of their illness. Find out by asking, for instance, "How are you processing this situation?" or "How is your spirit dealing with all of this?" How would you refer them to a specialist or counsel them about these issues yourself?

2. Identify a patient you're caring for whose illness is at least in part related to their own choices or behavior. Show them grace and acceptance. Treat them warmly. Encourage them to look forward, not backward. When it will help, tell them that God is all about second chances.

3. Identify a patient who is experiencing spiritual distress. Practice spiritual care by using one of the interventions described in this chapter.

4. Identify a patient you're caring for who is a spiritual nihilist or a moral legalist. Help awaken and encourage their spirit using the methods described in this chapter.

6

Healing and Repentance

A MAN WHO ATTENDED OUR CHURCH asked me to arrange a time when he could meet with the church leadership board to pray for healing. He had been diagnosed with a serious illness over a year previously and had had a disappointing response to treatment. Our board was accustomed to praying with sick people, following the process described in the epistle of James, and I told him I was happy to make the arrangements. But he was taken aback when I asked how his relationship with God was doing and whether he was practicing repentance. "What does that have to do with my health?" he asked.

"I'm not saying that you're somehow responsible for your illness," I told him. "We live in a broken world," I continued, "and we suffer because of that. But the Bible says that repentance can be part of the pathway to healing that God provides." This idea was new to him, and he was reluctant to discuss it. He subsequently came to one of our meetings, where we prayed together with him for healing but without mention of repentance.

The word *repentance* may sound old-fashioned and out of step. Yet we healthcare professionals regularly urge our patients to repent—to turn from unhealthy habits and embrace new ones. We do so because we understand that practices such as smoking, excessive alcohol use, and eating unhealthy diets are bad for our patients. Similarly, the Bible portrays repentance as both preventative medicine and a path to healing. In this chapter we'll look at the discipline of repentance and how it can lead both us and our patients toward health.

WHAT IS REPENTANCE?

The Hebrew word translated "repent" is commonly also translated "turn" or "return," and the Greek word means "a change of mind."[1] Repentance is more than feeling sorry. It involves changing direction. Imagine that you are driving to an unfamiliar destination and take a wrong turn. Repentance involves recognizing and regretting that you've gone the wrong way and turning around. Our patients who stop eating fast food and increase their intake of fruits and vegetables have repented of bad dietary habits.

I grew up understanding that repentance was a standard component of prayer. Yet for me repentance seemed to be an endless loop of confessing my failures, promising to try harder, and failing again the next day. My patients seemed better able to achieve positive change in their lives than I was. After all, some of them were able to break their unhealthy habits, but I found that there was no bottom to the bucket of my own shortcomings. I would revert to old habits or discover new ways in which I needed to change. I felt like a real-life Sisyphus, the mythological Greek king who was forever condemned to push a rock uphill only to have it roll to the bottom and have to start all over again. Was there more to it, I wondered, than that? If I miss the mark just as often today as I did yesterday, or last year, or a decade ago, what is the point of repentance?

I've come to realize that repentance is more than regret and correction. This description of repentance is missing the main thing that makes repentance Christian. Christian repentance is relational. It's an interaction with God. In fact, Christian repentance is primarily about recognizing and responding to God's presence. It's because of him that we are able to change.

Sometimes I best repent when I don't intend to. For instance, I was recently with a group of healthcare workers singing praise songs together. A few were singing with hands raised, rocking back and forth. One was dancing in place. I'm a less emotive person, and I was standing still with my hands at my sides. As my mind filled with the truths about God that the lyrics expressed, my emotions moved. My voice began to wobble, and I had to stop singing. I bowed my head, listening to the music and sensing God all around me, my eyes suddenly moist. His graciousness and love were so close. It was obvious in that moment that I am human and he is divine, that I fail but he never does. In his presence I tasted my smallness and his majesty. The best and only thing to do was to give myself to him all over again. Repentance happened not because I had intended it but because I was with God.[2] For days afterward that experience echoed through my prayers, lifting me up.

At other times repentance comes to me quietly, when I'm alone. When my workday is done, an episode from earlier in the day may come to my mind as I'm commuting or when I have time at home to reflect. It may be a clinical success I enjoy reliving, a decision I would now make differently, or an interaction I did not fully understand. As the scene replays, I view it from a new and unexpected angle, the perspective of God's Spirit within me. I see something of his pleasure or his sorrow or his purpose in that episode that I missed completely at the time. As I see an event through Jesus' eyes, I may be grateful for his provision in that moment—or I may realize that I did not resemble him, and may regret the way I acted. I experience his sadness, and I tell him so. I make the sometimes painful decision to set things right. I ask his Spirit to be more active in me during busy times, directing my steps as I take them. Only then does the peace that I had vaguely sensed was missing return to me. This sort of repentance is not a chore. It is a gift.

Repentance is our only pathway to God (see Is 30:15; Prov 1:23).[3] Whether it comes through worship, reflection, or the routine and dutiful practice of the daily discipline of prayer, repentance is a necessary personal response to Jesus. It's a requirement for citizenship in his kingdom (Mt 3:8; 4:17; Lk 24:47; Acts 2:38). Christ-followers regularly repent. It is the way we begin with God. The movement at the core of repentance is a turning toward God, a rediscovery of his presence—and the humble posture and honest self-appraisal that result. Repentance is not a lonely struggle up a mountain. It is repeatedly returning home. As we focus on God, he equips us.

This way of thinking about repentance can shift our attention from the past to the future. On a recent Monday morning I drove to work having slept poorly the night before. After parking my car in the lot, I sat behind the steering wheel, closed my eyes, and recognized that God was close. I prayed, "Lord, I confess that I don't have what it takes to be patient and loving with people in clinic today unless you do your work in me. Please fill me with your Spirit." I was silent for some moments, sensing God's response. That encounter with God reverberated through my clinic, changing how I approached my patients and colleagues.

As a healthcare professional I find it easy to stop practicing repentance. I am used to being in charge at work and taking care of problems. I know I'm good at what I do. It's uncomfortable to meditate on a less flattering view of myself, and it can be hard to slow down enough to realize God's presence. I find it easy to omit repentance from my daily schedule, which is busy enough as it is. But I've paid a personal cost for skipping repentance. I end up carrying burdens I could be transferring to God's shoulders—burdens of human suffering and responsibility. And my professional confidence, untempered by the humility of repentance, can morph into impatience and arrogance, negatively affecting the people I work with, live with, and take care of. It's ultimately in my best interest to regularly practice repentance. It's a path that leads to the fruitfulness and fulfillment God provides.

> I've paid a personal cost for skipping repentance. I end up carrying burdens I could be transferring to God's shoulders—burdens of human suffering and responsibility.

REPENTANCE AND HEALTH

Jesus portrays repentance as preventative medicine. He does so when commenting on the untimely death of people killed by a collapsing building, the sort of sudden and tragic event that still occurs today. He says, "Those eighteen who died when the tower in Siloam fell on them— do you think they were more guilty than all the others living in Jerusalem? I tell you, no! But unless you repent, you too will all perish" (Lk 13:4-5). Jesus begins by correcting the misperception that injury and death are meted out in response to the weight or number of our shortcomings. Those who died were not especially bad sinners, particularly deserving of judgment. They were like the rest of us. Their deaths therefore serve as a cautionary tale. Jesus offers a radical lesson for us to take away from this tragedy: "But unless you repent, you too will all perish." In the verses that follow he explains, using a parable, that we all fall short and all deserve death. The reason we're still alive is that God is patient with us. His patience gives us an opening, an opportunity to repent and be fruitful (Lk 13:6-9; see also Jer 18:8; Ezek 18:30-32; Amos 5:4; Rev 2:5). But that opportunity will not be available to us forever. We are all living on borrowed time. Elsewhere in Scripture God says, "Those whom I love I rebuke and discipline. So be earnest and repent" (Rev 3:19).

Repentance is preventative medicine because it remedies a life-threatening state of affairs.[4] We saw in the last chapter that sickness may in some cases be a form of divine discipline, a wakeup call. Here Jesus teaches us that the untimely suffering of others is also a wakeup call for us. Repentance is our healthiest response to the vicarious suffering we experience when we care for sick and injured people.

We healthcare professionals inevitably tell ourselves a narrative about the illnesses of the people we care for. Confronted with the suffering of a fellow human being, we may assume (as Jesus' listeners did) that they were destined for their affliction in a way that we ourselves are not. We all fear death, whether we realize it or not, and we often defend ourselves from that fear by denying death will come to us. Surely some combination of my patients' genes, exposures, and life choices explains why disease has befallen them and spared me! This way of thinking may hold some probabilistic truth, but Jesus teaches us that it is a dangerous misinterpretation of our patients' predicament. We are all equally deserving of untimely sickness and death.

Our healthiest response to the troubles of others is repentance, not denial. "There but for the grace of God go I." This distinctively Christian response to suffering can change our clinical approach: as our subconscious denial of our own inevitable death recedes, we're better able to be fully present with suffering patients. Indeed, an attitude of personal repentance may in part account for the prominent role of Christians in the historical development of hospitals and hospices.[5] It may sound difficult or even impossible to respond to our patients' suffering with an attitude of personal repentance. Our natural inclination is to deny that suffering will one day come to us also, instead of acknowledging that we too are destined to die and dependent on God. But when we do respond to the suffering and death we witness with repentance, not denial, the fear of death loses its psychological grip on us, and we can experience remarkable freedom (more on how this works in the next chapter).

REPENTANCE AND HEALING

When sickness is a wakeup call, the correct spiritual response is repentance. For instance, David writes about the health effects of taking his lieutenant Uriah's wife for his own and plotting Uriah's murder. He describes wasting and chronic fatigue as the results of his unconfessed sin: "When I kept silent, my bones wasted away . . . my strength was sapped as in the heat of summer" (Ps 32:3-4; see also 2 Sam 11–12). Confession and repentance led to forgiveness and marked the start of his healing.

But the Bible suggests that repentance is always a good idea when we're sick, regardless of whether our illness has any link to our own shortcomings. Here's how James portrays this idea:

> Is anyone among you in trouble? Let them pray. Is anyone happy? Let them sing songs of praise. Is anyone among you sick? Let them call the elders of the church to pray over them and anoint them with oil in the name of the Lord. And the prayer offered in faith will make the sick person well; the Lord will raise them up. If they have sinned, they will be forgiven. Therefore confess your sins to each other and pray for each other so that you may be healed. (Jas 5:13-16)

James teaches us that life events should prompt spiritual responses. Trouble reminds us to pray. Happiness leads us to praise. Sickness prompts us to confess our sins to each other and to seek the presence and prayer of wise Christians. Note that communal confession and prayer are an ordinary part of the Christian response to illness. Confession, out loud, to a pastor or a trusted and wise friend, can have transformative power in our lives. Repentance and prayer for healing are not reserved for times when we think our own sin has led to sickness or when medical treatments have failed.[6]

Why is repentance a routinely helpful response to illness? Thinking holistically, illness reminds us to

> The Bible suggests that repentance is always a good idea when we're sick, regardless of whether our illness has any link to our own shortcomings.

attend to all aspects of our health, including our relationship with God. A healthy spirit can have a positive impact on physical well-being, whereas spiritual problems can negatively affect bodily health (see chapter three). Repentance is therapeutic, especially for the soul and spirit, because it removes barriers between us and God, allowing us to transfer our worry and distress to him and experience his power and peace in return.[7] Repentance starts with the recognition of God's presence and includes elements of honesty, humility, dependence on God, awareness of our own inadequacy, and readiness to change. These all align us with our Creator and open us to his influence. This posture positions us for healing.

REPENTANCE IN CLINICAL PRACTICE

Repentance can increase our resilience and the fulfillment we get from our work. Here are some practical means of experiencing its benefits:

Practice repentance yourself. Many of us spend our days with sick people, yet we manage to deny that illness and death are coming to us also. But the burden of our repeated exposure to sickness and death takes a subconscious toll that can surface in our lives as emotional exhaustion, anger, lack of empathy and job dissatisfaction. I'm often tempted to skip past repentance and ask God directly for solutions to these issues, only to find that they weigh just as heavily on me afterwards. For me, a personal posture of repentance before God is a necessary part of regaining my balance and experiencing God's work in my life.

Bring repentance to work with you. We know ourselves to be effective and capable healthcare professionals. We are confident in our knowledge and skills, as we should be. There is joy in fulfilling our purpose by using our power for good, as God intended for us in Genesis 1. Yet it's easy for us to increasingly know ourselves as gods of our day-to-day worlds and to lose sight of the reality that we are broken and undeserving individuals. The inevitable result is that we become spiritually cold. There are diagnostic signs of this condition: if you care a lot about what other people think of you, if you get angry easily, if it's been a while since worship brought you joy, or if the gospel bores you, you may be allowing your professional identity to supplant your identity as a child of God.[8]

We best thrive in healthcare when our confidence goes hand in hand with humility, when we are conscious of our limitations and unhelpful tendencies, when we're ready to learn. How is it possible to know ourselves as both capable and flawed, confident and incomplete, skilled professionals and children of God? For a Christian, it often starts with recognizing God's presence in our workplaces and humbling ourselves before him.

I aim to pray whenever washing my hands at work, in the brief moments when I'm alone with my own thoughts before interacting with a patient or colleague. Sometimes, after seeing a sad case, my short prayer is, "Lord, you've favored me, and I don't deserve it." At other times, thinking about my next patient, I pray, "Lord, you know far more than I do. Please use me for good in this patient's life."

I also aim to pray when I'm unsure of the best thing to do. Maybe I'm looking at my next patient's test results or dealing with something unexpected in the middle of an interventional procedure. My best option in those moments is not frustration, anger, or looking for someone to blame. My best response is to relax into my faith: to pause and feel God's presence, to tell him I need help, and to ask him for wisdom in the middle of my workflow.

Encourage repentance. The statement "You should repent" is good advice for all of us, but it's usually not the best place to start with your patients! Repentance is about truly encountering God, so encouraging our patients to turn to God is often a good place to begin. The approach you take to encouraging patients to seek God will vary based on their cultural context, your particular work setting, and the spiritual history that you've already obtained from them. If you are working in a Christian healthcare facility, in a culture where belief in God is the norm, speaking directly about repentance and involving a chaplain in patient care may be your routine— although, for patients suffering from religious struggle, challenging them to repent without first responding to their spiritual alienation may backfire. On the other hand, if you are working in a secular context, in a culture that is increasingly detached from spirituality, cues from the spiritual history will help you decide whether a conversation about spiritual health will be productive. In either case, some patients have emotional barriers to faith that will have to soften in the face of our skill, compassion, and service to them before a conversation about their spirituality will be helpful. Assessment of the patient's spiritual condition precedes spiritual intervention.

The sidebar shows examples of how to start a conversation about spirituality that may be relevant to some patients and practice situations. Unlike spiritual history-taking, these often come toward the end of a patient encounter, when we're framing a treatment or management approach. It's often best to start with a question, giving patients the option to either discuss their spiritual health with us or else deflect the topic. Questions also reveal to what extent our patients are open to improving their spiritual health.

Sample Questions That Introduce the Topic of Spirituality

"We've already talked about a plan of treatment, but I know that illness affects many different areas of life. How is your spirit doing? How can I encourage you (or help you) with that?"

"What's going on in our lives can affect our treatment success. What's going on in your life these days? Would you like to talk about how you're doing emotionally, mentally, or spiritually?"

"You mentioned that faith used to be part of your life. When a health crisis comes, some of my patients say that God sees them through it. Are you interested in reconnecting with your spiritual side? What do you think the first step would be toward that?"

"In my experience, healthy relationships are an important part of overall health. That includes relationships with key people in your life—how are those relationships doing? How about your relationship with God? What steps do you think you could take to begin to connect/reconnect with God?"

"I sense that your spirit is suffering. Have you considered looking for spiritual support in a time like this? What's worked for you in the past? Can I suggest some practical steps?"

"Stress can really magnify health problems. What kinds of stress are you experiencing? What resources do you have to help you deal with stress? Do you have spiritual resources available that help you?"

Some patients may question the relevance of these sorts of questions to their medical care. The data linking spiritual practices and physical health, and the practice guidelines of authoritative healthcare organizations, detailed in chapter three, justifies our interest in our patients' spirituality.

Some of our patients may be inclined to curse God because of their ill health. Others may be disappointed with him, as though he's failed to keep his promises, and some may reason that they deserve better from him. But the spiritual pathway to healing runs through repentance, not anger, disappointment, or entitlement (Rev 16:11). We must respond carefully to our patients when these issues surface, resisting the inclination to offer a quick fix. Sometimes our role is to point to spirituality as a resource in difficult times, on the basis of our own experience, the experience of other patients, or the data we reviewed in chapter three. At other times we can model a healthy approach to God by praying a lament with our patient, as described in chapter nine. Some patients will be ready for this. For others, though, our best initial response is to listen with compassion, acknowledge their pain, and pray silently for wisdom. Our patients must know that we realize the complexity of their experience. This keeps the door open for future conversations when spiritual care might be offered.

Use effective strategies to encourage spiritual health. Consider how you regularly challenge patients to repent for the sake of their health: for example, to improve their diet, start exercising, or quit smoking. What approach do you take? Berating and lecturing are ineffective strategies for encouraging life change, and a judgmental attitude can raise barriers. Broad statements such as "You have to lose weight," unaccompanied by specific helpful strategies, are also ineffective. Evidence-based methods for helping our patients accomplish positive change include discussing the relevance of life change to the patient's situation; setting specific, measurable, attainable, relevant, and time-bound (SMART) goals; identifying potential barriers and addressing them directly; encouraging self-monitoring, including a log of relevant daily behavior; and asking for a commitment to small, discrete steps toward a goal.[9] Building a therapeutic alliance, presenting facts, telling true stories, providing treatment resources, and following up all have a role in helping our patients turn away from unhealthy habits toward healthy ones.

Many of the same strategies apply when it comes to encouraging our patients to invest in their spirituality—whether they're coping with a serious illness, undergoing a major intervention, or seeing you for a health maintenance consultation. Help patients who are interested in spiritual health set specific, attainable goals and identify small, discrete action steps they can take toward those goals. These might include seeking forgiveness from God and others, reconnecting with their faith community, reading and meditating on a text such as Psalm 23 or one of the Gospels, practicing gratitude, talking with a pastor, or praying about their illness. Include a spiritual diagnosis (such as "spiritual distress" or "desire for enhanced spiritual well-being") in your problem list. Follow up with them about these elements just as you would with other aspects of health.

> Help patients who are interested in spiritual health set specific, attainable goals and identify small, discrete action steps they can take toward those goals.

Enjoy responding to questions about spirituality. We may feel flat-footed when a patient looks to us for spiritual encouragement or guidance. In fact, this may be why we avoid mentioning spiritual matters with our patients in the first place. When you have the opportunity to respond to a patient's questions about spiritual health, you don't need to have all the answers. It's typically wise to lead not with theological statements but with your own experience—to talk about what God has done in your own life or the lives of other patients you've cared for. Your patient may be struggling to cope with new limitations, or in turmoil and longing for peace, or wrestling with despair, or looking for more in life—all of which you may have experienced at some point. Besides sharing anecdotes, you can offer resources, such as Bible passages, books, podcasts, or online videos that address your patient's situation, or you can refer your patient to a spiritual professional who can answer their questions.[10]

FOR REFLECTION

1. Describe whether and how you practice repentance, and the effect it has on your spiritual life and your professional life.

2. In what ways might an attitude of personal repentance change a Christian healthcare worker's interactions with their patients? How might it increase our resilience?

3. Do you think repentance can lead to healing? Does it always? In what sense is repentance therapeutic when physical healing doesn't occur?

4. In your context, how might you encourage your patients to turn (repent) toward God?

IT'S YOUR TURN

Perhaps you find repentance discouraging or pointless—or maybe repentance is something you've never applied to your work. It's time to try a new approach and discover the change it can make. Pick one or more of these exercises and work on them this week:

1. Make time to repent before work. Christian repentance is primarily an encounter with God. It is a posture more than an activity. Acknowledge God's presence by reading Scripture or singing a worship song. Pray Psalm 19:12-13 or Psalm 51:1-12 and personalize the verses. Sometimes repentance focuses us on particular shortcomings, but it is always a humble response to God's presence.

2. Try repenting forward: before your workday starts, tell God about the ways you are likely to fall short today and ask for his Spirit's help. Then touch base with him about it, in brief and silent prayer, in the middle of your workday or shift.

3. When you are caring directly for a suffering patient, try offering a brief silent prayer of repentance and thanksgiving: "God, you've blessed me with health. I don't deserve your goodness to me, but I'm grateful. Thank you." This sort of prayer can change how you relate to suffering patients and the fulfillment you find in caring for them.

4. Find opportunities to help your patients connect the dots between their physical and spiritual health. This doesn't mean attributing your patients' sickness to sin. It means reminding them that they're more than bodies, or mentioning that health has emotional and spiritual dimensions and asking how these are doing. In most healthcare contexts we do this by asking questions. Review the examples mentioned in the latter part of this chapter.

7

The Fear of Death

ONE MORNING I GOT A CALL from a resident working in the intensive care unit. "Do you remember Mr. Silva?" he asked me. "I do," I responded. "He had a gastrointestinal problem I treated a couple of years ago." "Well, he's been in the ICU for almost two weeks now," the resident said. "He was admitted with a large stroke and pneumonia. He remains unresponsive and is still on a ventilator. Our team thinks it's time to withdraw care, but his family doesn't agree. Would you come by and talk to them? They specifically asked for you." "I'd be glad to," I said.

That evening I stopped by the ICU. As I logged on to Mr. Silva's electronic medical record, I thought back over the few conversations we'd had. He and his wife had seemed wary of doctors. I had tried to encourage them. I had also taken a basic spiritual history.

His wife was at his bedside, and I greeted her. I sat down, and we talked. She asked whether there was anything more that could be done. I told her that I had reviewed his medical record and discussed his care with the ICU team. Medically speaking, there was nothing more to do. "I know he has faith in God," I said. "Tell me about that." She told me that they often attended a local church. "Is faith an important part of his life?" I asked. "It is," she responded.

"Miracles can happen, but he's had setback after setback," I said. "Maybe God is saying that it's his time." She was silent. I asked whether prayer would help, and she said yes. I held his hand and prayed for both of them. A couple of days later, I learned that care had been withdrawn, and he had died.

Many of us struggle to find helpful ways to interact with our patients about death. For some of us, death painfully exposes the limits of our craft. Others of us have not reconciled ourselves to our own mortality. The topic uncomfortably reminds us that we are not exempt. Despite all evidence to the contrary, we tend to assume that health is for us a permanent state of affairs, and we're often stunned when we hear that we have a serious diagnosis. Pastor Tim Keller, writing about his diagnosis of pancreatic cancer, said, "[My wife and I] expected some illness to come and take us when we felt *really* old. But not now, not yet. This couldn't be; what was God doing to us?"[1]

The prospect of death is frightening, and the fear of death can have a major but unrecognized influence on our lives. Conversations with our patients about death come easiest when we have a holistic view of personhood, a willingness to ask about the spiritual side of life, and are not ourselves under the subconscious sway of the fear of death. Otherwise, we may not be able to adequately communicate with our patients and their families, and support them as they face life's final enemy. That's why I've more than once been asked to mediate end-of-life conversations between a patient (or their family) and their care team. In this chapter we'll frame a biblical understanding of death, consider how the fear of death affects our culture, our patients, and ourselves, and describe how our own death anxiety influences our clinical practice. We'll then consider how we can keep the fear of death from blunting our professional satisfaction and subconsciously controlling our lives.

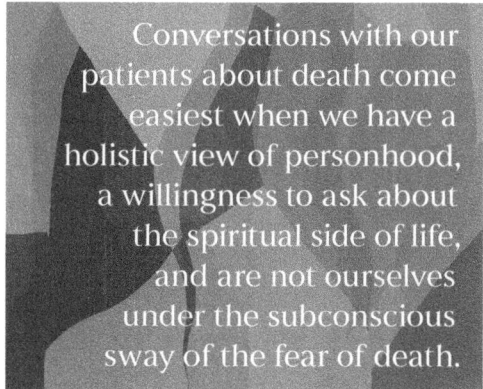

> Conversations with our patients about death come easiest when we have a holistic view of personhood, a willingness to ask about the spiritual side of life, and are not ourselves under the subconscious sway of the fear of death.

A BIBLICAL VIEW OF DEATH

Death is sometimes described as a natural part of the circle of life, but the Bible portrays death as our enemy (1 Cor 15:26). We were not originally created to die—we were made to last. In the Genesis account, it seems that Adam and Eve were not intrinsically immortal beings, but as long as they had access to the Garden of Eden's tree of life, their lives could persist (Gen 2:17; 3:19-24). Their act of disobedience and their banishment from Eden made death an inevitable part of their lives and ours. Death and decay are the sad result of a world skewed by sin, and our lives often end prematurely and painfully.

Does God determine the length of our lives? David, writing about how God formed him and knew him in his mother's womb, says, "All the days ordained for me were written in your book before one of them came to be" (Ps 139:16)—implying that God foreknew every aspect of his life, including its length. Scripture also gives us examples of people whose time on earth ended when God so decided.[2] On the other hand, the Bible sometimes depicts human choice and apparent happenstance leading to death.[3] Both God's sovereignty and human agency seem to play a role, and these factors need not be mutually exclusive.[4] Regardless, for Christians, death is about God's intimate knowledge of us and the meaning of the arc of our lives.

Job describes how disease made him long for death because it would relieve his suffering (Job 3:2-22). Jonah, in despair, asks God to end his life (Jon 4). God deals gently with both of them. Rather than granting Jonah's request or scolding him, God addresses the anger and turmoil in Jonah's soul. He shows Jonah that his anger is selfish, and that his life is not all about his own comfort and desires. It does not appear to be wrong to ask God to end our lives. However, he may deal with the root cause of our request rather than granting it.

Death is the most difficult and stubborn opponent we face. But Jesus, in returning from the dead, "has destroyed death and brought life and immortality to light" (2 Tim 1:10; see also 1 Cor 15:22; Heb 2:9). He is our pioneer, and by the power of God we too will be physically resurrected.[5] For Christians, death is not the end of life. In his poem "Time," George Herbert writes that death, once an executioner, is now a gardener, transplanting us to a better place.

THE FEAR OF DEATH

Fear of death encompasses fear of pain and suffering, fear of the unknown, and fear of extinguishment and loss. It is perhaps the most fundamental human fear, and it has some positive consequences: it can give us prudence in the face of physical risk and reluctance to end our own lives. However, the fear of death often has unfortunate and underappreciated influence on modern life. The author of Hebrews says that people are "held in slavery by their fear of death" (Heb 2:15), and Paul writes that death reigns over us (Rom 5:14-17). This means that our apprehension of death rules us and strongly influences our behavior.

Death was a more familiar part of daily life for people in biblical times than for most of us today: lifespans were shorter, medical care was rudimentary, and most people would have witnessed others die in childhood or the prime of life. However, the fear of illness, aging, and death continues to influence human behavior.[6] Some of us deny death by celebrating youth and doing everything we can to appear young. Others are reminded by their approaching retirement of the nearness of death and experience "retirement anxiety."[7] Still others become obsessed with signs of possible illness and fixate on medical care as the way to escape death.

Many of us rarely think about death because the psychological mechanisms of avoidance and denial shield us from the terrifying reality that death is certain, close, and beyond our control. But the fear of death nevertheless affects our lives and cultures. Social scientist Ernest Becker asserts that fear of death is a fundamental factor determining the structure of human civilizations and is "the mainspring of human activity," motivating our behavior. He posits that we respond to our innate, subconscious fear of death by pursuing either literal immortality (via religion or technologies such as cryopreservation) or symbolic immortality (through offspring, fame, wealth, influence, or accomplishment).[8]

> Many of us rarely think about death because the psychological mechanisms of avoidance and denial shield us from the terrifying reality that death is certain, close, and beyond our control. But the fear of death nevertheless affects our lives and cultures.

According to Becker, we buffer death anxiety and derive our self-esteem by believing we meet or exceed our own worldview's expectations and values, in contrast to others.[9]

Subsequent empirical research has supported these ideas. Subconscious awareness of death alters electroencephalogram (EEG) patterns and heightens our tendency to compete with others.[10] When primed with the idea of death, people are more likely to think well of themselves, opt for confrontational or violent solutions to conflict, become angry or judgmental, favor negative and prejudicial stereotypes, trenchantly defend their own values, become stingy, and experience prolonged grief after loss.[11] When reminded of their own mortality, judges set higher bonds for defendants, and jurors respond more critically to evidence.[12] Fear of death manifests as ageism, a term for discrimination based on age. The fear of death heightens our tendencies to be judgmental, impatient, aggressive, prejudicial, defensive, and critical.

Among healthcare professionals, our own death anxiety influences our clinical practice. For instance, among nursing students, fear of death is associated with a negative attitude toward the care of dying patients, and nurses with a greater subconscious fear of death are more likely to experience professional burnout and leave nursing practice.[13] Death anxiety was associated with lower subjective well-being and poorer sleep quality among doctors working during the Covid-19 pandemic.[14] When breaking bad news to their patients, oncologists with greater personal fear of death have more emotional difficulty, pay less attention to their choice of words, and make less eye contact with their patients.[15] When caring for the dying, we may prioritize relief of symptoms over human presence, and they may die alone.[16]

Our patients' feelings about death can drive their approach to healthcare. Health-seeking behavior and health anxiety may be motivated by the fear of death, and worries about death are associated with the presence and severity of psychological problems including depression, anxiety, and somatic symptoms.[17] Fear of death also influences patient preferences regarding end-of-life care.[18] Death anxiety is common among family members of sick patients and correlates with their need for spiritual support.[19]

FAITH AND THE FEAR OF DEATH

Does religious faith ease the fear of death? Empirical studies have come to conflicting answers, and a clear relationship has not emerged.[20] But despite the absence of a consistent reduction in their fear of death, religious adults experience less anxiety and depression and greater psychological well-being than others.[21]

One way to synthesize these findings is to conclude that the prospect of suffering and dying is frightening for people regardless of their religious beliefs, but faith protects us from the sway that the fear of death can hold over us. This returns us to the biblical book of Hebrews, which says that Jesus is able to "free those who all their lives were held in slavery by their fear of death" (Heb 2:15). Notice that Jesus frees us not from the fear of dying but rather from bondage to that fear.[22]

The prospect of dying can be fearful for persons whose identity is rooted in Christian faith, but that fear does not own us. We can live and act free from the subconscious influence that the fear of death exerts on life. How is that possible? It has to do with habitually recognizing the presence of Jesus and aligning with him.

Jesus came to earth "to shine on those living in darkness and in the shadow of death, to guide our feet into the path of peace" (Lk 1:79). His presence dispels the shadow that the fear of death otherwise casts over us. As we recognize him in real time, our allegiance to him supplants other influences in our lives. When we align ourselves with Jesus, our trust in him overtakes our fear of death, and that fear loses its power over us (Heb 2:15). Our union with Christ, who has defeated death on our behalf, is our passport to life and peace (see Mt 4:16; Lk 12:4-7; Acts 2:24; 2 Cor 1:22; 5:15; 2 Tim 1:10; Heb 2:17).[23]

My problem is that my self-identity shifts. I'm a child of God and a follower of Jesus, but I'm also a husband, father, son, brother, physician, friend, jogger, gardener, consumer, and citizen. When days and weeks go by without touching base with God, my allegiance to Jesus frays. My status as God's child has waning influence on my thoughts and actions. My beliefs are unchanged, but my spirit dims. The shadow of the fear of death starts to creep over me. I catch myself becoming impatient and critical of others, and work seems increasingly routine and technical. Intellectual assent to Christian doctrine is not enough to free me from slavery to the fear of death. I need to live in the presence of Jesus. It's the warm radiance of his presence that frees me. He puts me on the path of peace.

The apostle Paul is a remarkable example of a Christian who was free from slavery to the fear of death. In his letter to the Philippians, penned while he was under house arrest and awaiting trial in Rome, he writes:

> I eagerly expect and hope that I will in no way be ashamed, but will have sufficient courage so that now as always Christ will be exalted in my body, whether by life or by death. For to me, to live is Christ and to die is gain. If I am to go on living in the body, this will mean fruitful labor for me. Yet what shall I choose? I do not know! I am torn between the two: I desire to depart and be with Christ, which is better by far; but it is more necessary for you that I remain in the body. (Phil 1:20-24)

He wrote these words facing the possibility of imminent death. He felt death anxiety and hoped that his courage would be sufficient when the time came but also looked forward to what would come after death. Far from being enslaved by his fear of death, Paul writes that "to die is gain." How could he genuinely feel that way? He identified strongly with Jesus. His life purpose was to work for Christ, and he knew that his life would not end until his work was done. He affirmed that when he did die, he would immediately be in the presence of Jesus (2 Cor 5:8). His overarching aim was to know Jesus, not only in life but also in the process of dying, "becoming like him in his death, and so, somehow, attaining to the resurrection from the dead" (Phil 3:10-11).[24]

The subconscious fears that commonly drive people lose their power over us as we identify with Jesus.[25] We live in service to the one who has defeated death on our behalf. As we regularly choose union with him, we become free from the grip that the subconscious fear of death holds over many people. We become less judgmental and defensive, and better able to focus on and appreciate others. The freedom we experience in life expands our horizons.

The practical choices we make can help align us with Jesus and combat the power of the fear of death in our lives. Sometimes this involves developing habits of Bible reading, prayer, or Scripture memorization. At other times it helps to stop dwelling on things that might otherwise buffer our death anxiety: our professional title, social position, bank or investment balances, belongings, accomplishments, or the praise we've received from other people, none of which actually shield us from death. When we're generous with our time and resources, we combat the stinginess that the fear of death provokes. When we give others the benefit of the doubt, we move away from the judgmental attitude the fear of death imposes.

We can also deny the power of the fear of death by stepping away from the comfort and security people around us prize. For instance, my wife, Janet, and I left a rewarding life in America and took up work in sub-Saharan Africa in the summer of 2019. Some of our friends were mystified by our decision. Why give up the recognition, safety, and prosperity that our American situation provided? We explained that, over several years, we had felt God nudging us to move on to something new. In following God's direction and shedding many of the secular things that buffered our death anxiety, we experienced a renewed sense of freedom in life. Six months after moving to the horn of Africa, we were challenged by the arrival of the COVID-19 pandemic. People around the world were dying from coronavirus infection, and we didn't have access to treatments available in the United States. We tried to act wisely, taking precautions to limit our exposure to the virus—but we also affirmed that we were where God had led us, and we chose to stay on. That decision reinforced our dependence on Jesus and further contributed to the freedom we've experienced.

THE FEAR OF DEATH IN HEALTHCARE PRACTICE

Some of us regularly come face to face with death in our clinical practices, while others of us do not. Regardless, the fear of death lurks in the background of many clinical scenarios that we all commonly deal with. An identity rooted in Jesus, not our work, shields us from the discouragement and dissatisfaction that the fear of death can impose on us. It also makes us better caregivers. Here are four practical ways to experience freedom from slavery to the fear of death in your practice:

Recognize that fear of dying is universal. Jesus was human, and he experienced anguish as death approached (Lk 22:39-44; Mt 26:38). For many of us, faith does not eliminate that turmoil. Don't be surprised when believers and nonbelievers alike struggle with pain or are anxious when death is near. In his distress Jesus sought comfort from the attentive presence of his disciples. As healthcare workers who have walked with others along this stage of the human journey, we have the privilege of being present with our patients and of easing their pain and suffering.

Human companionship is important to dying people. Rather than succumbing to our own fear of death and looking away from the dying, we can be present for dying people ourselves. As people approach death, they often focus on their spirituality and life's significance, and we can be sounding boards for their thoughts and concerns. We can ask about their life story. We can take (or retake) their spiritual history and learn (by asking questions) whether they have unmet spiritual needs. Christian patients may be encouraged by reading 2 Corinthians 4:7-18, where Paul writes about Jesus' victory over death for us and the inward renewal we can experience even as our lives are failing, or 1 Corinthians 15:35-58, which describes the resurrection from the dead and the hope this gives us. Some of our patients intellectually assent to Jesus' victory over death but have not yet chosen to align themselves with him and experience the freedom that brings; they may want to give their allegiance to him. Others are searching for hope, and we can (if they so desire) share with them the hope we've found. For almost all of our patients, no matter their views on faith, the caring presence of other human spirits is a primary source of comfort as death approaches.

Take a balanced approach to preventative health. Medical approaches to disease prevention are God's good gifts to humanity, and we encourage our patients to adopt evidence-based approaches that can prevent serious illness and prolong productive life. However, medicine is not able to release people from bondage to the fear of death, because death remains inevitable despite the best medical care.

Some of our patients may become obsessed with signs of possible illness and fixate on medical attention as a subconscious response to their fear of death. With such patients we may have the opportunity to help them cope with the force that is driving them. Often the best initial approach is to seek insight by asking questions about their responsibilities and goals, close relationships, and experiences with death and spirituality—all without minimizing their medical concerns. Referral to a wise counselor can be helpful.

At its best, preventative medicine includes consideration of soul health and spirit health, which are necessary components of wellness. To thrive—to live in a state of shalom—we must be free from slavery to the fear of death. Faith has the power to heal our patients in ways that medicine cannot.

Understand that our patients' spiritual health is essential to their well-being. People can experience psychological well-being and human flourishing when the fear of death no longer masters them. This is a strong reason to encourage our patients' spiritual health, because faith offers freedom from bondage to the fear of death that medicine can't provide. This is true for all our patients, no matter the severity of their health issues.

For patients whose current healthcare problems are routine and curable, our conversations naturally focus on the medical or surgical issue at hand. It may be appropriate to encourage the patient to take a step back and consider their overall body, soul, and spirit health, particularly when stress, lifestyle, psychological issues, troubled relationships, or overwork are amplifying or contributing to their medical problems. A routine health issue may be a wakeup call for a patient who is struggling emotionally, relationally, or spiritually.

With patients whose diseases are chronic, complex, or life threatening, conversations about our mortality often best occur in the setting of an established relationship. They require the patient's permission as well as respect, calmness, and encouragement from the healthcare professional. It may be appropriate to begin with a statement such as, "I want to understand what you're thinking about where your medical care is going." Atul Gawande describes three questions he asks patients with incurable disease: What are your biggest fears and concerns? What goals are most important to you? What tradeoffs are you willing to make, and what ones are you not willing to make? (The last question takes into account the benefits and adverse effects of various treatment options.)[26] These questions help us understand our patients' hopes, fears, and goals and are a good place to start but don't clarify their spiritual beliefs and concerns. We can add open-ended questions about soul and spirit health, as discussed in detail in chapter three, for instance, "Is faith important to you? Is it shaping how you think about this situation?"

Recognize that we are healthiest when our identity is rooted outside our profession. When we know ourselves primarily as Christ-followers and daily choose to serve him, we experience freedom from slavery to the fear of death. Our perspective shifts from our own self-esteem toward the well-being of others, our prejudices loosen, and we better understand others. We gain deeper emotional resources, enabling us to care for people without falling quickly into compassion fatigue. We become better caregivers: more fully present with our patients, better able to truly listen, coach, and guide them, and less prone to discouragement ourselves.

How do you know whether the fear of death holds sway over you? Here are some indicators: if you have little interest in patients you can't cure, if you're uncomfortable caring for dying patients, if you're quick to (perhaps silently) judge and criticize others, if you have difficulty accepting criticism, or if you're quick to become angry, the fear of death may have undue influence in your life. The remedy is to align yourself with Jesus day by day. The habit of daily experiencing union with Jesus is key to flourishing as a Christian healthcare professional. Make time in your schedule to pray, meditate on Scripture, and worship.

How do you know whether the fear of death holds sway over you? Here are some indicators: if you have little interest in patients you can't cure, if you're uncomfortable caring for dying patients, if you're quick to (perhaps silently) judge and criticize others, if you have difficulty accepting criticism, or if you're quick to become angry.

FOR REFLECTION

1. Secular and religious healthcare professionals agree that it's important to talk about death and dying with patients facing poor prognoses—but these conversations often don't happen. Why do you think that is? When and how would you begin a conversation with a patient about death and dying? Consider the practical examples mentioned in this chapter.

2. What is slavery to the fear of death (Heb 2:15), and how is it different from fear of death? What impact does this have on how we live? In what ways is slavery to the fear of death apparent around you today?

3. In what ways do Christians fear death? Not fear death? Read Philippians 1:20-26; Luke 22:39-46; and Acts 2:24.

4. How might you offer comfort against the fear of death? How (if at all) will this differ with patients who do or do not share your beliefs?

IT'S YOUR TURN

We healthcare workers witness death, and our subconscious fear of death can drain our joy and steal our career satisfaction. Freedom from slavery to that fear can revitalize us. Regularly aligning ourselves with Jesus is key to the benefits this chapter talks about. Here are practical ways to get started:

1. Take a personal inventory. To what extent are you influenced by the subconscious fear of death? Apply the indicators in the last paragraph of this chapter to yourself.

2. The fear of death can show up in our lives as anger and intolerance of others. How do you respond to your own feelings of anger, fear, or irritation? If you've been dealing with these dark emotions recently, ask Jesus for the light of his presence with you in real time, guiding you into the path of peace (Lk 1:76-79).

3. Most of us avoid thinking about death, especially our own deaths. In your prayer life this week, thank Jesus for your health. Tell him that you know you'll die eventually and that your hope is in the resurrection he promises. Acknowledge that, in the long run, it's

what you do for him that matters in life. Thank him for his Spirit within you, and ask him to free you from slavery to the fear of death. Return to this sort of prayer when you have firsthand experiences with death and dying.

4. One practical way to loosen the grip of the fear of death is to practice generosity. By giving our time or resources to others, we counter the stinginess that the fear of death provokes. When we give to others, we shrug off a scarcity mindset and adopt an abundance mindset rooted in God's abundance toward us.[27] Be generous this week by giving financially to a person or cause you believe in, or make a point of giving other people the benefit of the doubt, or be generous with the time and attention you give to your patients, family, and friends.

PART 3

Suffering

the compassion fatigue that builds as we care for suffering people. While there are various responses to compassion fatigue, including psychological education, resiliency training, and structural workplace changes, research shows that personal spiritual practices can mitigate compassion fatigue—practices we'll explore.[4] Job's story shows that there is much about suffering that we don't understand and can't control, but we can choose how we respond to it. Healthy patterns of spiritual response can restore our resilience, compassion, and joy. Unhealthy responses can compound the fatigue we feel as we care for suffering patients and manage difficult situations.

> Job's story shows that there is much about suffering that we don't understand and can't control, but we can choose how we respond to it.

JOB'S STORY

Job was a man who lived in the ancient Near East. The book of Job is a poetic masterpiece and one of the oldest texts in the Bible.[5] It can be divided into three main parts: an introductory account that describes how Job came to suffer (Job 1–2), an extended middle section composed mainly of dialogues between Job and his friends about his suffering (Job 3–37), and a climactic finale in which Job interacts directly with God (Job 38–42). In this chapter we'll focus on the first part of the book, which describes how Job chooses to respond to suffering with integrity.

The story begins by describing Job as a prosperous person with a large family, huge wealth, and a great reputation. He was a blameless, morally upright man who feared God (meaning God was often on his mind, and he approached God with reverence and awe) and shunned evil. Job would offer sacrifices for each of his adult children after they had parties in case they had sinned. Job was authentic: what you saw was who he really was. There were no skeletons hidden in his closet. The congruence over time of his public life and private life, of his actions, mind, and heart, is called his *integrity*.

Early in Job 1, the scene shifts from Job's earthly life to a heavenly court, where angels present themselves to God. One day Satan comes, and God asks him, "Have you considered my servant Job? There is no one on earth like him, blameless and upright" (Job 1:6).[6] Satan responds that Job respects God only because God takes care of him, prospering him. He asserts that Job's allegiance to God is not a sign of integrity: instead it's part of an unspoken bargain, a quid pro quo in which loyalty is traded for blessing. Satan proposes a test. He suggests that if God will "strike everything" Job has, Job will curse him (Job 1:11). God responds, "Very well, then, everything he has is in your power" (Job 1:12).

In due course disaster comes from multiple directions, killing Job's children and destroying his wealth. Job mourns, but he doesn't curse God; he worships God instead. The next time Satan comes to the heavenly court, God again mentions Job, saying, "He still maintains his integrity, though you incited me against him to ruin him without reason" (Job 2:3). Satan responds, "Now stretch out your hand and strike his flesh and bones, and he will surely curse you to your face" (Job 2:4). Subsequently, Job is afflicted with a painful, chronic health condition. Job's illness may have been hyperimmunoglobulin E syndrome, pellagra, leprosy, elephantiasis, or syphilis.[7] His symptoms include physical wasting, fever, insomnia, anorexia, difficulty eating, skin lesions, and chronic pain (Job 6:7-30; 7:4, 14; 19:20; 30:30; 33:19-21). The physical changes he experiences are so extensive and unpleasant that people avoid him and his friends no longer recognize him (Job 2:12). Job's suffering is so severe and persistent that he wishes he had never been born (Job 3:1-19; 10:19).

What is the *why* of Job's illness? The text makes clear that his sickness is not due to any wrongdoing on his part. Satan raised a fundamental challenge regarding the nature of religious practice: the integrity of human faith and worship is being tested. Yet it doesn't seem right that Job should suffer as a test case. We know God is love and that his love encompasses all of his creation, and so we want to believe that he has a beneficial purpose in mind for Job himself.[8] Yet that purpose, if it exists, is not mentioned in the first part of the book.[9] Moreover, the events taking place in the heavenly court are completely hidden from Job. He has no inkling about why he is suffering. Our patients are often similarly in the dark about the meaning and significance of their suffering, and so are we.

JOB'S INTEGRITY

Job passes the test that has been set for him. He does not curse God, as Satan had predicted he would and as his wife urges him to do. He chooses instead to maintain his integrity.

Job keeps his integrity by continuing to affirm truths about God and himself, truths he held to before God withdrew his blessing and disaster came his way. His worldview—his understanding of the world in general and his life in particular—doesn't shift with his circumstances. He affirms that God is in charge of the world and has control over his life, and that God has the right to give people blessings and difficulties. These truths are the pillars of his response to suffering. When his wife says, "Are you still maintaining your integrity? Curse God and die!" Job responds, "Shall we accept good from God, and not trouble?" (Job 2:9-10). Instead of cursing God, Job says, "The LORD gave and the LORD has taken away; may the name of the LORD be praised" (Job 1:21). He places responsibility for his calamity at God's feet, but he doesn't question God's purposes or character. Nor does he attempt to resolve the philosophical problem of suffering. He chooses instead to worship God and accept what God has brought him. The text tells us, "In all of this, Job did not sin by charging God with wrongdoing" (Job 1:22).

The first chapters of Job make clear that God is sovereign, meaning he has kingly authority and control over all of his creation. Theologians debate whether God intends or merely permits suffering, but in either case God is in charge and could have prevented Job's suffering if he chose to—just as he has the power to prevent the suffering we and our patients experience.[10] The text also demonstrates that suffering's ultimate cause can be completely hidden from us. Furthermore, Job has no control over the events that overtake his family or the illness that consumes him. The only thing he controls is his own response to suffering, his own integrity.

CHOOSING INTEGRITY IN RESPONSE TO SUFFERING

How can Job's decision to maintain his integrity inform our responses to the suffering we witness and the compassion fatigue we experience? Here are five practical applications to our own healthcare practices:

Remember that God is in charge. It's difficult to care for human suffering at close range day after day, particularly when we have inadequate solutions. In these times I find it helpful to remember that God is ultimately responsible for my patients' suffering—I am not. My job, of course, is to relieve suffering and restore health, and I pursue these goals for my patients to the best of my ability. But God is the one who determines the outcome of my efforts. He is in control, and disappointing outcomes— even when seemingly random from the biomedical point of view—are under his discretion.

When adverse events happen at work, we have an obligation to stick by our patient, continuing to care for them with excellence. We review what happened, and if we've failed to meet a standard of practice we must acknowledge that and learn. Adverse events force us to confront our own limitations, to admit that there is a lot we don't understand, and to reexamine our own purpose in healthcare. We can give the emotional burden of these situations to God. He is the one who determines the results of our work. Emotional freedom enables us to treat our patients with clarity and compassion. The next time a patient of yours suffers a poor outcome, tell God about it. You'll be better able to respond to the situation.

Choose prayer. As compassion fatigue builds, we might respond by growing distant from God, but our healthiest response is to pray instead. Research shows that prayer increases the satisfaction we derive from caring for others and makes us less vulnerable to compassion fatigue.[11] In response to taxing clinical scenarios, we can pray in a way that makes God a part of the equation. Here are some examples of prayers that may forestall compassion fatigue: "Father, Ms. Agbani [is suffering, or being difficult, or not responding to treatment]. I know that you care about her, and that you've put me here to care for her. I'm [unsure what to do for her, or not feeling much love for her right now]. I need your help." "God, give me wisdom as I take care of Mr. Garcia. You're in control. Show me how to treat him. We're both trusting in you for solutions." "Father, I'm running out of compassion and feeling irritable. I need your comfort myself. You're my source of caring and strength. Thank you for your goodness in my life." In response to these sorts of prayers, God's Spirit comforts our spirits, and his caring concern recharges our caring concern for others (2 Cor 1:3-4, which we'll return to in more detail in chapter twelve).

Choose congruence. It's easy to compartmentalize our professional and personal lives, our practice and our faith. Integrity implies that our various roles—healthcare professional, child, sibling, parent, spouse, friend, colleague, child of God—are one whole cloth, without contradictions. Don't check your faith at the door to your workplace. Bring God to work with you. And don't leave workplace issues behind when you go to church, meditate on Scripture, or pray. Talk to God about them and seek his perspective.

> In response to taxing clinical scenarios, we can pray in a way that makes God a part of the equation.

Choose worship. Integrity is fundamentally a matter of our hearts, not our minds. For some of us, exposure to the suffering of others leaves us with a mind that is theologically correct but a heart that is distant from God. After all, we don't understand why he allows suffering to continue, and our gratitude, love, and awe of him may fade. But a cold heart impoverishes our spirituality and drains our compassion. Worship is often our best path to integrity because it too is rooted in our hearts. We were made to worship. If the image of God in us is an angled mirror, reflecting God's care into the world, it also reflects in the other direction, "summing up the praises of creation" back to God in worship.[12] When we worship, we assign ultimate value to God, not to ourselves, and we affirm that he is our shepherd, our loving father.[13]

For our own sakes we can choose to respond to the reality of suffering with worship, like Job did, especially when worship doesn't come easily. Choosing to worship when God seems distant and the outlook is bleak strikingly affirms the integrity of our faith. Find ways to worship that revive your spirit and make them a part of your routine. Use worship to combat compassion fatigue by renewing your connection to God and aligning yourself with him. Listen to or sing worship music during your commute or at home before and after work. Try worshiping briefly during your workday, in moments of prayer or song that honor, praise, and give thanks to God.

Choose love. Consider the three statements from the start of this chapter, all of which Scripture affirms: God is all-powerful. God is all-loving. Suffering is real. Of these, God's love gets the least attention in the first section of Job. In the middle section of his book, Job goes astray as he loses sight of God's love. It's easy for us and our patients to lose sight of God's love too. When we're suffering from compassion fatigue, we can choose to experience God's love by turning toward him instead of turning away. More on that in the next chapter.

FOR REFLECTION

1. What instinctive responses do people have to the suffering of others? To what extent do these reactions influence our decision to become healthcare professionals, and our choice of healthcare role and specialty?

2. Read aloud the first two chapters of Job. How does Job's story challenge popular conceptions of God, for instance that God is not responsible for human suffering or that we get from him what we think we deserve?

3. Sick Christians are sometimes counseled that unconfessed sin is causing their illness. Others may tell them that suffering is never God's will. In light of Job's story, how would you respond to these common ways of thinking about suffering?

4. Are you experiencing compassion fatigue? An online assessment tool called ProQoL can help you sort out whether the satisfaction you get from caregiving is outweighed by emotional fatigue. Answer the "compassion satisfaction" subscale questions[14] and discuss your results with a friend.

IT'S YOUR TURN

Your faith gives you resources to combat compassion fatigue and increase your joy in your work. Put these resources to use. Here are ways to get started:

1. When irritation or hurry are welling up in you at work, slow down for a moment with your next patient to learn something about them

as a person, as described in chapter one. Recognizing the whole person before you, made in God's image and eternal, can reset your perspective, invoke God's presence, and renew your caring concern.

2. Worship is a bulwark that can mitigate compassion fatigue. Make worship part of your workday routine. Find a playlist of praise songs to listen to during your commute or during your lunch break. Use music to remember God and honor his goodness.

3. Put a Bible app on your phone and use it to read psalms during breaks at work. Use them as templates for prayer. If you've lost sight of God's majesty, pray Psalm 8. If you need his care, pray Psalm 23 or Psalm 121. If you're surrounded by troubles, read Psalm 34. If God seems to be absent, pray Psalm 13. If you're finding it hard to praise God, pray Psalm 103.

4. We are trained to respond effectively to patients' physical suffering, but we sometimes overlook their spiritual suffering. After asking a patient how they are doing and hearing about the status of their physical symptoms, ask how their spirit is doing. Pause to give them space to answer. If they share a spiritual struggle with you, you don't have to offer a solution right away. Thank them for telling you. Pray about it.

9

Lament

BILL ARDILL IS AN AMERICAN SURGEON who lived in West Africa for decades, caring for countless patients and training many African colleagues. One night he heard a noise coming from his neighbor's home. When he went to investigate, armed robbers shot him at close range with a sawed-off shotgun. Amazingly, he survived. He was evacuated to Europe and the United States, underwent multiple operations, and endured medical complications. Despite treatment, he continued to suffer from pain and disability, compounded by despair.

Bill writes, "It seemed that as I was walking along with God, he stuck out his fist and smacked me in the face and knocked me flat on my back." He says that he became

> quite depressed at a perceived absence of God in my painful moments. . . . I thought I was not a steadfast Christian, was not a strong father, and had not projected triumph, praise and victory through my suffering. Rather, I had been beaten down completely by the pain and loneliness to a point of despair and complete discouragement. It was humbling, terrifying and depressing.[1]

How, in practical terms, can we continue relating to God when we ourselves are suffering—or when compassion fatigue leaves us weary and ill-equipped to respond to patient needs and difficult clinical scenarios? It's easy to doubt God's power or his love. It's easy to stop trying to relate to him at all. For me it can be hard to read Scripture, pray, and worship when my days are full of the difficulties of others, and even when I practice these disciplines they can seem mechanical and joyless. It can be even more difficult for our patients to relate to God while suffering. A friend of mine stopped coming to church after his illness was diagnosed. "Why," he asked, "would I praise a God who let this happen to me?"

In this chapter we'll contrast Job's response to suffering, as shown in the middle section of his book, with a type of response called lament. We'll see that a healthy response to suffering chooses to engage directly and repeatedly with God, affirming both the reality of suffering and God's powerful and loving character. Lament gives us a pattern for prayer that we can use in response to the suffering of our patients and our own compassion fatigue. Lament—as opposed to simply asking God to fix a problem—is key to recovering hope and peace in difficult situations, in both our personal lives and at work.

> Lament—as opposed to simply asking God to fix a problem—is key to recovering hope and peace in difficult situations, in both our personal lives and at work.

JOB'S MISSTEP

The extended middle section of Job contains a series of dialogues between Job and his friends, who wrongly believe that Job's calamity is a punishment from God. While Job maintains his innocence, they counsel him to confess the wrongdoing that they believe led to and propagates his suffering. As his sickness progresses and his isolation worsens, Job becomes bitter. He affirms that only God can save him (calling God "my Redeemer"), but he also asserts that God has turned against him and oppressed him (Job 19:6-12). Using courtroom analogies, he gives evidence of his innocence (Job 31) and portrays God as an unjust judge who has delivered a verdict against him before the trial even starts (Job 10:1-17).[2] Mark Talbot calls this Job's "misstep:" he maintains that God is powerful but loses sight of God's steadfast, unfailing love (Hebrew *hesed*) and stops believing that God is beneficent.[3] Job challenges God for an explanation, but at the same time recognizes that God, in his sovereignty, holds all the cards. He talks about God more than he speaks directly to God. He feels powerless and falls into despair.

Some of our patients follow in Job's footsteps. God's love seems to be absent from their circumstances, and they resolve the conundrum of suffering by concluding that God doesn't care, has given up on them, or is actively punishing them. Like Job, they may favor talking about God over interacting with God directly. They may drift away from God, abandon their relationship with God, or doubt his existence. In all of these ways their spiritual health can suffer.

As we respond to the suffering of others, we may come to the same conclusions about God. We too can stop believing in our hearts in God's steadfast love. I know this from personal experience. As the burden of responsibility of healthcare work builds within me, I can keep going through the outward habit of church attendance but stop relating to God in prayer, meditation, or worship—maintaining a form of godliness but missing out on its power.

LAMENT

Laments are prayers in response to adversity. They are found throughout Scripture, particularly in some of the psalms written by David. His youth was punctuated by a series of severe challenges that he overcame by trusting in God, and his adult life was marked by an unshakeable, vivid belief in and reliance on God. He was not perfect, and his shortcomings are laid out in detail in biblical accounts. Yet he always returned to God and is called "a man after God's own heart" (see 1 Sam 13:14 and Acts 13:22). David's laments were usually written in response to danger, sickness, or distress.

Lament offers us a template for prayer and meditation when we're burdened by the suffering of others. The key elements of lament include (1) turning to God while suffering, (2) bringing our problem to God, (3) remembering God's love and past faithfulness, (4) asking boldly for help, and (5) choosing to trust God.[4] Let's consider each element in turn.

Turn to God while suffering. This is the key initial step on which other elements of prayer in times of suffering hinge. Sometimes it seems easier to avoid God, even while going to church, than to focus our minds on God and speak with him. But talking directly with God about our situation is a prerequisite to a healthy spiritual response to suffering. David instinctively turns to God for comfort in times of turmoil. Instead of turning to God, Job often speaks about God—not to seek shelter in him but to question God's character, to argue his case, or to ask God to leave him alone (Job 10; 13; 19). Whether you are suffering yourself or fatigued by the suffering of others, choose to turn to God and talk to him about it.

Bring your problem to God. David freely describes his distress to God: "Out of the depths I cry to you, LORD" (Ps 130:1). "My heart pounds, my strength fails me, even the light has gone from my eyes" (Ps 38:10). "Heal me, LORD, for my bones are in agony. My soul is in deep anguish. How long, LORD, how long?" (Ps 6:2-3). In Psalm 22, David describes an episode of severe physical and emotional distress in detail. He vividly tells God what he is experiencing. We can too.

David, like Job, doesn't hesitate to attribute his situation to God: "All your waves and breakers have swept over me" (Ps 42:7). "Day and night your hand was heavy on me" (Ps 32:4). "You lay me in the dust of death" (Ps 22:15). We too can attribute our situation to God. He has allowed—or even intended—our situation to occur, and we can tell him so.

It may seem unnecessary to tell God what we're enduring, since he already knows. Yet the Bible repeatedly demonstrates that describing our situation to God is an important step toward experiencing his comfort. When we tell our story in prayer, we encounter the sympathetic ear of Jesus, our advocate. We open the door to experiencing his presence with us in real time. Our predicament has significance and purpose, which he understands even though we don't. As we tell him our woes, we sometimes gain his perspective on our circumstances.

Remember God's love and faithfulness. Bringing the past to mind can be key to finding hope in the present. In his laments, David reflects on who God is and what he has done in the past, both in the events of his own life and in the history of his people. He remembers times when God's mercy and love supported him and, sure that God is unchanging, translates these past events into the present. For David, remembering is more than mental recall. It is the past influencing his present choices and behavior.[5] Historical and theological truths are anchors that give him hope that God will save him from his current predicament.

In a virtuous cycle, each blessing David receives from God enriches his history with God and strengthens his certainty that God is a God of steadfast love, who will never abandon him (Ps 118:8-14). Job, on the other hand, looks back wistfully at his past and comes to believe that God intends to crush him (Job 10:3-8). But the God of the Bible is not fickle. His love for us does not ebb, nor does it depend on any virtue of ours. David's choice to remember God's love and faithfulness can be our choice also.

The crucifixion of Jesus demonstrates the depth of God's love for us. Out of love, Jesus took on all of our suffering.

> [If we've been treated unfairly] then on the cross, to our astonishment, we see God the subject of unjust suffering, weakness and death. . . . If we've lost a loved one, to our astonishment we look at the cross and see the Father losing his only son. Or, if in our pain, we are screaming out "Why, God?" we look at the cross, and there is Jesus screaming out "Why, why?" He suffered everything we have ever suffered.[6]

He endured what we endure and more in order to win victory over suffering and death for us.

When you're tired of caring for the suffering of others, think of times when God has met your physical, emotional, and spiritual needs, or those of your family, friends, patients, and community. Recall the ways he's provided for you. Remember occasions when God's love embraced you. Tell him about those times and the aspects of his character they reveal. Recall also that Jesus experienced what you're experiencing. He has endured it with you and for you.

Ask boldly for help. Some Christians hesitate to ask God for practical help. David had no such qualms. He writes: "You are my strength; come quickly to help me. Deliver me from the sword, my precious life from the power of the dogs. Rescue me" (Ps 22:19-21).

Sometimes reluctance to pray for healing reflects pride or a fatalistic worldview. Other times it exposes a mistaken belief that God, who is spirit, has no influence over physical things. We believe in a God who created our reality and who has the power to change that reality. David repeatedly asks God for help in dire situations, and so can we.

I tend to ask God for help without first telling him my story or reflecting on his past goodness to me. Often the results seem vaguely unsatisfactory. He can seem distant and unmoved. Telling him my problem and remembering his past goodness bring his presence into focus and prepare me to receive whatever he has for me in the moment.

Trust God. Mark Voegrep writes that this is the destination of all lament.[7] In threatening situations, David actively chooses to trust God with his future. For David, trust leads to hope: "I wait for the LORD, my whole being waits, and in his word I put my hope" (Ps 130:5). Often David's expressions of trust turn into anticipatory praise and a vow to glorify God in the future (Ps 22:22-24; 35:7-10).

Job intermittently expresses trust in God, even though God seems to be his unloving adversary. His determination to trust in God, even though he takes no comfort from his faith, marks the high point of his struggle with suffering in the middle portion of his book. During his own ordeal Bill Ardill, quoted at the start of this chapter, read Job. He writes, "The verse that haunted me the most was 'Though He slays me, still I will trust in him.' . . . That was my goal—to renew and re-establish my trust in God in spite of or through my circumstances."[8] Expressing trust in God sometimes brings almost immediate comfort. Other times it can be years until that comfort comes. Yet in either case, choosing to trust in God is an act of integrity and hope.

It's easy to pray for help without dwelling on God's loving character and without expressing trust in him. Yet both of these elements are key to a healthy spiritual response to suffering, and when we omit them we may miss out on the peace and hope that prayer can bring. A spoken commitment to trust God, to wait hopefully for him and to praise him, galvanizes our spirits and aligns us properly with him.

Cycle between elements of lament. Mark Talbot writes that the psalms of lament "show us how to breathe." In his distress David exhales and inhales elements of lament. Talbot describes phases of breathing: telling God about our distress (exhaling), remembering truths about God (inhaling), asking boldly for help (exhaling), and choosing to trust in God (inhaling again).[9]

Think of a woman in labor using breathing techniques to cope with pain. One breath is not enough: the pain is still there, and she repeatedly responds with additional breaths. In a similar way, when we're suffering, turmoil and distress intrude on our prayers. When trouble was foremost in David's mind, repeatedly interrupting his focus on God, he kept praying, vocalizing his distress, and reflexively responding with remembrance, request, or trust. In many of his laments he cycles between his own complaint and affirmation of God's character, between asking for help and relying on God. There is no required order to the elements of lament. David's laments "coach us to keep calling on God, to keep addressing him, even if that means complaining or protesting. In short, we must keep breathing."[10]

Lament can be therapeutic in a way that simply asking for help is not. It energizes our spirits by renewing our connection to God—a conduit through which peace and hope can flow. It reminds us that God is present and can be trusted. The acronym TREAT helps me remember the components of lament: tell God your complaint, remember God's love and faithfulness, ask God boldly for help, and trust in God. Respond to the suffering of others, or your own compassion fatigue, by TREATing it.

> The acronym TREAT helps me remember the components of lament: tell God your complaint, remember God's love and faithfulness, ask God boldly for help, and trust in God.

LAMENT IN THE BIOMEDICAL PARADIGM

The lament form may seem familiar to healthcare professionals because it parallels modern healthcare interactions. The difference is that medical interactions are between a patient and a healthcare provider, not a sufferer and God, and we're on the receiving end of the lament. The elements of lament are all present in medical consultation: the patient speaks directly to their healthcare professional, describing their complaint. Their general knowledge and past experience suggest that we are effective healers. Their very presence with us is a request for help. They place their confidence in us (sometimes even telling us, "I trust you") and believe that we will effectively care for them.

What happens to healthcare professionals when we're repeatedly given broad latitude and Godlike discretion in the lives of our patients? On the one hand, our privileged position is essential to the effective performance of our profession. On the other hand, playing God takes a toll on us. Our shoulders are not that broad. When things are going well, the thrill of playing a Godlike role may shift our self-identity increasingly to our professional persona and away from dependence on God himself. We may grow distant from him, and, as our identity shifts, we may increasingly act superior to people in our private and community lives. Our family and friends may perceive us as unloving and arrogant. And when things are not going well for our patients, a habit of bearing all responsibility ourselves—of assuming that the buck stops with us—can put unbearable stress on us, compounding the burnout and compassion fatigue we experience.

Our profession's self-conception has changed dramatically over the decades. In the past healthcare professionals often assumed a Godlike role, making healthcare decisions for their patients and bearing the consequences, in the belief that this was best for their patients. This remains the case in some cultural contexts. However, in many settings the pendulum has swung in the other direction, with health professionals believing that their job is merely to offer their patients a menu of diagnostic and therapeutic options, providing information but putting the full burden of decision-making on the patient, shifting to them the weight of responsibility that we traditionally carried.

A biblical view of this issue lands us in between these two extremes. We are not God, and it's not best for us or our patients to act as though we were. We are also more than providers of information and technical skill. We show respect and help restore dignity to people who are suffering. We bring healing to God's creation on his behalf. We are embodiments of his love for people who are hurting. We are competent guides through healthcare's complexities, understanding our patients' anxieties and goals, sharing decision-making with them, and willingly accepting responsibility for their care.

How can we maintain this balance? We can best deal with our patients' laments by passing them on to God, using lament ourselves. We avoid playing God by acknowledging that God is the one who is all-loving, all-powerful, faithful, and trustworthy. When we affirm that God is present at the point of care and ask him for help in real time, his Spirit gives us comfort and wisdom, and his love and care shine through us to our patients.

LAMENT IN DAY-TO-DAY HEALTHCARE PRACTICE

As you deal with difficult clinical situations and the suffering of others, here are five practical ways to use lament for your own benefit while you're at work:

Keep turning to God. If you've stopped speaking directly to God on a regular basis, take this as a warning indicator, a flashing red light about your own spiritual health. Add up the number of times you stop even briefly to talk to God during the week. If you do this infrequently, this may be a diagnostic sign of a cold heart. Respond by making regular time in your schedule to pray, reflect on Scripture, or worship. Let these be times when you can give God your full attention, even if briefly.

When life doesn't make sense, wait on God. After experiencing suffering, we sometimes gain insight. Long after the trauma of his gunshot wounds, when he was once more practicing surgery, Bill Ardill wrote about himself and his wife, Dorothy: "Our faith in (God) was tested, our trust in him deepened, and our confidence in his love and sovereignty grew. . . . Although I do not want to revisit any of the painful moments of my past, I admit I have grown closer to God through them."[11] We wait on God by repeatedly telling him that our hope is in him and that we're waiting for his comfort, direction, and help. When we wait on God, we can ultimately reap a harvest of strength and peace.

Lament on behalf of your patients. Make a point of passing others' suffering on to God by means of lament instead of holding on to the weight of their suffering yourself. The elements of a TREAT prayer can be reduced to two breaths that fit into a busy workday. For instance, we can pray while logging on to an electronic medical record, while scrubbing before surgery, or when washing our hands between patients: "Lord, Ms. Patel is in distress. You are my strength—I'm trusting in you to help me take care of her." At other times we have the opportunity to pray with our patient, and can pray a lament on their behalf: "Father, we know that you're here, and that you care about Mr. Park. He is in pain [or feels weak, or is facing surgery]. You've had your hand on his life and have led him this far. I ask you to relieve his pain [or give him strength, or guide our hands during surgery] and restore him to health. We both trust in your love for us."

Include in your prayer an affirmation of God's goodness and an expression of trust in him. If we believe prayer is effective, then we can consider prayer a part of our therapeutic armamentarium. When we lament on behalf of a patient, the weight of their situation shifts onto God's shoulders.

Lament for yourself. Many of us are facing increasing levels of stress in our workplaces. Lament enhances our ability to cope even while we advocate for changes in the systems we work in. Instead of turning away from God, rely on your relationship with him by bringing your fatigue and dissatisfaction to him (1 Pet 5:5-7; Mt 11:28-30). Tell God what you're going through, remember his past faithfulness to you, ask him for wisdom, and trust in him.

Lament is a vehicle for affirming truths about our situation and about God. When we lament our view broadens: instead of thinking only of our circumstance, we remember that God is within earshot and we remind ourselves of who he is. If we choose to focus on him, lament can tune us to God's wavelength and prepare us to hear from him. In this way, lament may sometimes be an on-ramp to a new experience of God. More about that in the next chapter.

Choose love. Like Job, our patients can feel they're living in a universe from which love has disappeared. We may be the only embodiment of love they can see. But our stores of compassion are not bottomless. We best embody love over time, not by draining our own compassion, but by being conduits of God's love to our patients.

Situations of acute physical suffering are not usually the time to talk about spirituality or even take a spiritual history from our patients. We show compassion to suffering people by promptly and effectively treating their acute distress. When Jesus met a distraught widow getting ready to bury her only son, he chose to raise her son from the dead, without preaching (Lk 7:11-14). But even in these urgent situations we can speak simple, loving words, offer encouragement and reassurance, and mention our patient's courage.

In response to acute suffering, we can also demonstrate God's love by being present. The suffering of others can be hard to witness, and our human instinct may be to leave them as quickly as possible. By choosing to linger or return to the bedside, we embody the reality that God is near. We can show love simply by our attentive presence.

In other situations we demonstrate Christ's love by going the extra mile to solve an issue our patients are facing. Other times we draw out the image of God within them by taking an interest in their whole persons, as discussed in chapter one. With some of our patients we can speak of God's steadfast love for them and pray with them for help, peace, and hope.

The key to being a conduit of love in all of these scenarios is to recognize God's presence and ask him for help. By turning to him when we're fatigued, we give his Spirit the chance to renew us in the image of Christ (Col 3:10). We can become more like Jesus not only at church or while studying Scripture—we can become more like Jesus while we're at work, connecting with him in the middle of our workflow.

FOR REFLECTION

1. As he experiences suffering, Job loses sight of God's goodness. As healthcare professionals who often deal with the suffering of others, might we be prone to Job's way of thinking? How might this manifest?

2. Print out Psalm 86 and mark each of the elements of lament with a different color marker or pencil (telling God our complaint, remembering God's love and past faithfulness, asking boldly for help, trusting God). Notice how David cycles between elements.

3. How could the lament form help someone who is suffering? How could a TREAT prayer (either for ourselves or our patients) help Christian healthcare professionals who are at risk for compassion fatigue?

IT'S YOUR TURN

These exercises will help develop healthy responses to the depletion we feel as we care for others—responses that remind us of God's presence and love and mitigate compassion fatigue.

1. Resist the urge to quickly leave a patient who is suffering. Spend fifteen to thirty seconds with them beyond the time needed to accomplish your tasks. Sit down next to them. Look into their face. Hold their hand. Let your spirit be with their spirit.

2. Write out a lament on behalf of yourself or a patient, using the TREAT mnemonic: **t**ell God your complaint, **re**member his past love and faithfulness, **a**sk boldly for help, **t**rust in God. Pray your lament.

3. When you no longer feel caring concern for others, respond by praying brief laments for your patients or yourself. Always include an affirmation of God's goodness and an expression of trust in him.

10

When We Ask, "Why?" God Says, "Who!"

ETHAN HELM WAS FIFTEEN YEARS OLD when he was diagnosed with cancer. His adolescence was interrupted by invasive medical procedures, radiation treatments, and chemotherapy. He had to stop playing soccer. Kids at school made fun of his baldness. He suffered from headaches and vomiting. Worst of all, he learned the odds were against him. He knew that he might well die.

As he went through treatment, Ethan mastered the video game *Diablo*, becoming a sorcerer at the game's top level of difficulty. He was able to evaporate demons with fireballs and replenish his mana (his character's energy source) at will. Ethan describes his bedtime routine after hours of gaming:

> I climbed up the stairs from the basement, ate a bowl or two of Lucky Charms, and then went to my room to face my demons. I opened the door to my forest green painted walls, grabbed my Bible, crawled on my bed, and pleaded with God.
> "Why me, God? What have I done?"
> Demons surrounded me.
> Head under water.
> "How can a loving God permit suffering?" I thought of small bald children coughing in the waiting room, their parents staring at them,

uncertain of whether their child would live or die. "What crime has a two-year-old committed? What crime have I committed? Where is justice?"

I ran out of mana; I could cast no more spells.

Head under water.

I gripped my Bible and breathed deeply. "I don't have to believe in You."

I paused.

"There is no God!" I said, with immediate regret. The demons attacked. Defenseless, they hit me, and my life bar drained. Soon I would die.

Head under water.

I burst out of the water.

"God, I love you. Forgive me."

Eyes swollen and exhausted, I escaped from the demons with only a bit of water up my nose. Almost every night I fell into this pattern. After hours of killing demons, I'd run out of mana. Water covered my head as I wrestled with God. I never beat God, and He never left me, although sometimes it felt like He had.[1]

When I'm responding to suffering or stressed by difficult clinical situations, the question "Why?" can consume me. It's a natural question, aimed at the meaning of the circumstances I'm dealing with, but, like Ethan, I often find that there seems to be no satisfactory answer. Intellectually it can help to review the theology of suffering—its origins in Adam and Eve's disobedience, and God's plan to restore his creation at great cost to himself—but this may bring me little comfort in the moment or perception of a way forward. As I focus on *why*, the possibility of spiritual encouragement fades from view like a trail that peters out in a forest, leaving me at a standstill, frustrated and exhausted. Sometimes I camp out where the trail disappears. Other times I backtrack and find the right path, the response to the reality of suffering that leads me to peace.

In the middle section of his book, Job explores the cul-de-sac called *why*. Convinced of his innocence, and increasingly unsure of God's character, Job becomes eager to cross-examine God: to ask him to somehow justify the trouble he's experienced. Then, in the final chapters of the book, God speaks directly to Job. When God speaks, he shatters Job's expectations and our expectations too. In an unexpected twist, Job has a fresh experience of God that dramatically changes his perspective and creates the conditions for his healing.

It may surprise you to think that we too can have a fresh experience of God from a place of professional fatigue and discontentment. How does that work? Let's look at what God says to Job and how Job responds.

GOD SPEAKS

At the end of Job's remarks in the middle section of his book, he asks why God is silent, why he has brought calamity on him, and why he has not acted justly (Job 30:20-26). Several chapters later, after Job's friend Elihu has finished speaking, God answers Job out of a storm.

God's answer to Job's *why* at first seems to be no answer at all because he doesn't speak about the purpose or causes of Job's suffering. He doesn't mention the conversations in the heavenly court, described in the first part of the book, that apparently led to Job's calamity. Nor does he blame Satan. Instead of justifying himself, revealing his purposes, or directly resolving the philosophical problem of suffering, God instead talks about *who*: who he is and who Job is.

God starts with a question: "Who is this that obscures my plans with words without knowledge?" (Job 38:2). He goes on to illustrate the profound limitations of Job's knowledge and understanding. Although Job is among the most respected, influential, and literate persons of his time, God points out that he was not present at the start of creation, and he lacks insight into the dimensions, functioning, and future of the universe.[2] With sarcasm, God asks Job whether he knows how light originated: "Surely you know, for you were already born! You have lived so many years!" (Job 38:21). Furthermore, God demonstrates that he controls and sustains creation, and Job can't. "Can you bind the chains of the Pleiades? Can you loosen Orion's belt? . . . Can you set up God's dominion over the earth?" (Job 38:31, 33).

God then describes some of the ways in which he is intimately present and providing for his creation, far beyond Job's awareness. He asks Job, "Do you hunt the prey for the lioness and satisfy the hunger of the lions . . . ?" (Job 38:39). A lioness, of course, hunts for herself—but God arranges things so that she can catch and kill the proper prey, satisfying the hunger of her pride (Ps 104:21). Similarly, God describes his presence with a pregnant doe. She may seem alone as she suffers through labor and delivers her fawn in the wilderness, but God is there with her (Job 39:1-4). He provides wild donkeys with autonomy in a harsh habitat that suits them. He gives the ostrich both its speed and its foolishness: "God did not endow her with wisdom or give her a share of good sense. Yet when she spreads her feathers to run, she laughs at horse and rider" (Job 39:17-18). Through these examples, God develops a picture of nature in all its complexity, full of creatures he created, provides for, and cares about. He manages every aspect. He wrote the music, he made the instruments, and he conducts the symphony of life. Suffering is part of the score.

How is this relevant to Job? God demonstrates that Job is part of an incredibly large and diverse ecology, set within a universe God designed, delights in, and personally sustains. There is a vast

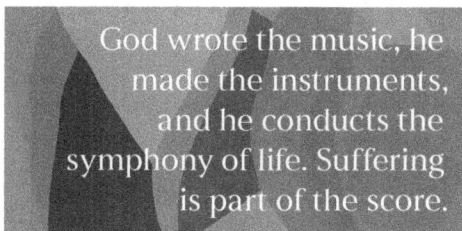

> God wrote the music, he made the instruments, and he conducts the symphony of life. Suffering is part of the score.

differential in perspective, power, and understanding between the two of them. Given his place in the created order, Job has no standing to question God's motives or actions. He lacks the insight and position to understand God's purposes or question God's fairness (Job 40:8).

God goes on to point out that Job can't save himself. He does not "have an arm like God's" (Job 40:9). He describes powerful animals (the behemoth and the leviathan) that Job can't tame. If Job is unable to control these beasts, why does he think he can successfully face off against God himself? God goes on to say, "Who then is able to stand against me? Who has a claim against me that I must pay? Everything under heaven belongs to me" (Job 41:10-11).

Although Job has recognized God's sovereignty—his kingly rule—from the start, God's statements demonstrate the basis for and magnitude of his sovereignty, as well as the extent of his caring concern. In comparison to God, Job is puny, his knowledge is scant, his power is weak, his intelligence is merely human, and his arguments are blind. He can hear a part of the symphony of creation, but he did not write the score. He does not know how the whole orchestra sounds or how the music will progress.

JOB RESPONDS

When God has finished speaking, Job replies:

> You asked, "Who is this that obscures my plans without knowledge?"
>> Surely I spoke of things I did not understand,
>> things too wonderful for me to know.
> You said, "Listen now, and I will speak;
>> I will question you,
>> and you shall answer me."
> My ears had heard of you
>> but now my eyes have seen you.
> Therefore I despise myself
>> and repent in dust and ashes. (Job 42:3-6)

There are several remarkable elements in Job's response. It is much briefer than his earlier dialogues with his friends. He doesn't repeat any part of his previous lengthy complaints, but he quotes God twice. He has a new understanding of both God and himself. And he reports a new experience of God that leads him to repent.

What was new about Job's encounter with God? It was direct in a way he had never experienced before. We can imagine that he had previously learned about God from the teaching and example of others, the evidence found in nature, and perhaps from sacred texts and religious ceremonies: "My ears had heard of you." But now he has had an intimate and unmediated experience of God, and he says, "My eyes have seen you." This doesn't mean that Job literally viewed God: the use of sensory language implies that the eyes of Job's heart encountered God directly and personally.[3] Think of a time when you spoke directly with a person after having repeatedly heard about them from others. Having met them, you know them in a way you never could have before.

The power of this experience causes Job to abandon *why* and dwell on *who*. The magnificence and power of God overwhelm him, and Job realizes how limited he is. He recognizes that he has no proper answer to the questions God asks him, no self-justification, and he regrets his previous questioning of God's character and purposes: "Surely I spoke of things I did not understand, things too wonderful for me to know." Job is awed, humbled, and acutely aware of his smallness. He realizes that the answer to the question "Why?" is beyond him. He despairs of his human limitations and wonders how he could have been so arrogant toward God.

A direct encounter with God causes us to instinctively recognize our smallness and ignorance in comparison to his grandeur and omniscience. That is why repentance was Job's immediate response to God's presence. Job repented of presuming that he deserved and could get answers from God.[4] Recall that repentance means turning and that Christian repentance is a relational act, triggered by and done in God's presence, that rights our relationship with him (see chapter six). Remember also that repentance is a posture that positions us for healing. In repentance we stop questioning, begrudging, or ignoring God and bow at his feet, in need of his mercy and focused on him. He is a God of steadfast love, who brings healing to our spirits—and oftentimes our bodies—as we repent before him.

In Job's case, healing came without his asking for it. Repentance was enough. The text tells us, "The Lord blessed the latter part of Job's life more than the former part," and he died "an old man and full of years" (Job 42:12, 17).

JOB'S EXPERIENCE AND OURS

Almost without our noticing it, Job's story gives us an answer to the philosophical problem of suffering. God is all-powerful, God is all-loving, and suffering is real. All three statements are true. The solution to their logical incompatibility is that our limited perspective, our embeddedness in time, and the smallness of our minds prevent us from unraveling the paradox. At best we can "explain why we can't explain suffering, understand why we can't understand it."[5] More importantly, the philosophical problem has become irrelevant to our response to suffering. *Why* is not what matters. *Who* is what matters: the magnificence of God and our response to him.

Is the sort of direct and immediate experience of God that Job had possible for us today? Yes, it is, if anything more so than in Job's time.[6] It's possible to experience God's presence in the valleys of life (Ps 23) or when we stand on literal or metaphorical mountaintops that give us glimpses of how vast and good God is—but also in the routine exercise of the Christian faith and in the middle of our busy workdays.

God is ready to communicate with us. He is spirit, and we are spirits made in his likeness who can relate to him. He is not distant: his Spirit dwells within us. But typically he doesn't clamor for our attention. There are means of tuning ourselves—like we would tune an instrument—to harmonize with God's Spirit. These include prayer, meditation, and worship.

I often enter prayer with an agenda and rush through it, leaving no room for response from God. Even lament, described in the preceding chapter, can seem like a one-way communication heavenward—but it involves affirming God's faithfulness and trustworthiness, and if we pause in prayer to appreciate God's character and remember his goodness we may become aware of his presence. For me, humming a praise song is a means of interrupting the train of my own thoughts and perceiving God's presence. Often it's a song I listened to before leaving home or during my commute, and it resurfaces in me throughout the day. For others, theological study—understanding the full story of creation, fall, redemption, and restoration—places suffering in context, shifts their focus to God, and brings the realization that "God has already told us these things are going to happen, whether we can explain them or not."[7]

During one dry spell in my own spiritual life, the Bible no longer seemed to speak to me. I would read a passage and find nothing but a reflection of my own thoughts. Out of frustration, I decided to try Scripture memorization, something I had not done for decades. When I was a kid, I would memorize an assigned verse on the way to church, recite it in Sunday school, and forget it by the time I got home. This time I decided to memorize slowly, hoping the verses would stick. I printed out Philippians 2, folded the paper so that it would fit in my pocket, and carried it with me. I regularly reviewed the verses when I jogged, slowly making progress. It took me a month to memorize the whole chapter. I started to see fresh applications of what I had memorized to my own life, so I kept going, slowly memorizing the whole book.

During this time I was one day struggling to achieve a good outcome for a patient during an interventional procedure. None of the usual maneuvers were working. It's easy in moments like this to become frustrated or angry or to look for someone to blame. But that day, words from Philippians 4 entered my mind, unbidden: "Let your gentleness be evident to all. The Lord is near. Do not be anxious about anything, but in everything, by prayer and petition, with thanksgiving, make your requests known to God. And the peace of God, which transcends all understanding, will guard your hearts and your minds in Christ Jesus" (Phil 4:6-7). I felt God's presence in real time and decompressed into the comfort of his presence. I thanked him for being there and asked him for wisdom. As I relaxed into my faith, God's peace filled me and gave me clarity, helping me best respond to the clinical problem I was facing. Since then, those verses have repeatedly resurfaced in my work life.

We can prepare ourselves for the premonition of God's presence by worship, prayer, study, or Scripture memorization. Doing so helps us discover him in new ways even when we're focused on the healthcare tasks at hand. It's possible to be at work and be with him, our spirit with his Spirit, sometimes communicating beyond words.

FINDING GOD IN DIFFICULT MOMENTS

We work in stressful professions. The stakes are high. The stress of repeated exposure to suffering, stubborn clinical problems, difficult patient personalities, and unexpected clinical events can lead us to a place of professional exhaustion and discontentment. Job's story shows us that, as we let go of *why* and focus on *who*, these times can be doorways to a fresh experience of God—at work, not at church—and an unexpected pathway to peace. Here are practical steps that can lead you to this experience.

> Job's story shows us that, as we let go of *why* and focus on *who*, these times can be doorways to a fresh experience of God . . . and an unexpected pathway to peace.

Remember that you control your response. We can choose to respond to the weight of clinical demands in many different ways. It is common to run low on personal resources, to feel irritation and fatigue, and to grow distant from God. The books of Job and Psalms signal us to turn to God for help with the weight of our work. When we turn to him with integrity, lament, and repentance we experience his comfort, love, and help.

Move past why. Rereading Job 1–2, I suspect that God had higher purposes for Job than the text states, purposes that somehow incorporated what was best for Job. But God doesn't need to justify himself to Job or to us, and his purposes in the difficulties we face often remain hidden or misconstrued by our attempts to discover them.

Partway through his ordeal, Ethan Helm, the video gamer I quoted at the start of this chapter, went on a weeklong trip with other pediatric cancer patients. He met another teenager named Martin, and they told each other their experiences, each of them sharing everything out loud for the first time. Ethan writes:

> When I spoke of my quarrel with God, Martin spoke boldly and powerfully. "God is more amazing than cancer is bad." I agreed. He then advised me, "Ethan, you can't do this without God. You need Him. You might not understand why things are happening, and that is okay, but you need to put your faith in Him. He will take care of you in one way or another." These words changed me. Instead of focusing on my anger with God, I put my faith in Him. I knew I could not do it without Him. Understanding He does not require, but faith He loves. After I did this, everything went better. My attitude, health and confidence all improved.[8]

Logic and scientific reasoning are at the core of our healthcare competence, and we must practice logically to practice well. But the logic of *why* can be inadequate to explain the meaning of difficult clinical situations or our own compassion fatigue. When that's so, our best response is to shift our focus from *why* to *who*, perceiving God's presence, relaxing into our faith, and trusting him in the moment. As we deal with the weight of our work this way, we trade frustration for clarity and peace. We become aware of God's comforting presence, and we're often better equipped to return to the clinical difficulty we're facing with new insights or fresh approaches to the problem.

Seek a fresh experience of God. When we're worn down, or feeling that we have little left to give to others, we can voice our complaint to God—often repeatedly. But our complaint is not a conclusion. Use prayer, Bible reading, memorization, and worship to tune yourself to God's frequency so that you can hear from him when you're burdened

> Our best response is to shift our focus from *why* to *who*, perceiving God's presence, relaxing into our faith, and trusting him in the moment.

or stressed at work. It may help to memorize Psalm 23 or to read Job 38–39, which remind us how vast God's purposes are and how much he cares for each individual creature in his creation. Affirm that his ways are beyond your understanding and that his ways are best. Acknowledge the magnificence of his power and the magnitude of his love. Sing to him. Ask God to reveal himself to you in a direct and personal way.

Rely on God. Our God is close to those who suffer, including us. He takes on our grief: "But you, God, see the trouble of the afflicted; you consider their grief and take it in hand" (Ps 10:14). He gives us strength: "So do not fear, for I am with you; do not be dismayed, for I am your God. I will strengthen you and help you; I will uphold you with my righteous right hand" (Is 41:10). We have no better choice than to turn to him as we care for our patients.

FOR DISCUSSION

1. In the face of suffering, does it make sense to affirm both that God is sovereign and that he is good? How can we account for the apparent contradiction in these propositions?

2. How, if at all, can you tune yourself to God's frequency—so that, when difficult situations arise, you're prepared to recognize his presence?

3. How might we, as healthcare professionals, follow Job's example in Job 42:3-6? How could this sort of response to the weight of our work increase the satisfaction we derive from our healthcare careers?

IT'S YOUR TURN

Is your world a little grayer when you've run out of professional bandwidth? Do the burdens you carry home from work take their toll on your family and social life or make you feel distant from God? Often these are signs that our workplace conditions need to change—but our personal spiritual practices also play a role in restoring our equilibrium. Try the following exercises.

1. Tell God about the aspects of your work that tax you the most. Maybe it's being responsible for other lives, dealing with death, the volume or nature of the work, your supervisor, or running out of caring concern for your patients or coworkers. Describe the situation in detail. Repent of your self-reliance and admit that you need his help. Before each work day or shift this week, ask his Spirit to remind you of his presence and to give you clarity and peace when work is stressful.

2. Use Job 42:2, 5-6, as a starting point for prayer. If it doesn't feel right to pray, "Now my eyes have seen you," ask for a fresh experience of God's presence. Find time to read Psalm 23 and consider what it says about difficult and stressful times, or Psalm 139:7-12, and reflect on what it teaches about God's presence in dark situations.

3. Over the next week, memorize Philippians 4:4-7. Recite these verses to yourself in the shower, while exercising, and at bedtime. Focus on the order of the words. Notice the role of thanksgiving in finding peace. Ask God to bring these verses to mind and give you a spirit of thankfulness at difficult moments of your workday.

PART 4

Good News

11

Healing and the Gospel

MY PATIENT WAS an intravenous drug user hospitalized with pneumocystis pneumonia. He was struggling to breathe, and while in the hospital he learned that he had HIV infection and AIDS. He had not graduated from high school, but he seemed savvy and tough, able to survive on the street in ways I could not. I thought we had little in common.

I made a point of sitting on the edge of his bed every morning during my rounds. I would look him in the eye as I was checking his pulse and ask him how he was doing. At first I got one-word answers. Gradually his oxygen requirements decreased, his dyspnea eased, and he started responding in full sentences. One day, expecting little, I asked him whether faith was a part of his life. He told me that, as a boy, his grandmother had taken him to church every Sunday.

I asked whether faith was important to him now. We were both silent for a moment. To my surprise, tears began to roll down his cheeks as he looked out the window. "I don't think God will take me back," he said.

"The good news is that God is all about second chances," I responded. "Look at the improvement you're making." I asked him whether he wanted to see a pastor from his grandmother's church, and he said yes.

The Christian good news, or gospel, contains a powerful message of healing, but for years I had trouble understanding it. Jesus' simple formulation of the gospel—"The time has come. . . . The kingdom of God has come near. Repent and believe the good news!" (Mk 1:15)–seemed obscure to me. It appeared to be missing the key element of the gospel that I had been taught, namely, Jesus' payment for my sin by the sacrifice of himself. Beyond that, I was unsure what the nearness of the kingdom had to do with belief in Jesus.[1] The pithiness of Jesus' statement made it all the more impenetrable, and the link the Gospel writers insisted on between this "good news" and the healing of disease (Mt 4:17-23; 9:5; Lk 4:18, 40-43; 7:12; 9:6) seemed tantalizingly opaque. Yet at work I sometimes saw physical healing and spiritual renewal occur together, as for the patient I just described. Was this coincidental, or did it reveal something about the gospel?

In chapters two and three we saw that our bodies, souls, and spirits are knit tightly together, threads in the eternal fabric of ourselves. By healing physical afflictions, Jesus showed that he saves not only souls but whole persons, bodies included. In this chapter we'll further explore the link between the gospel and physical healing. We'll find that the kingdom of God has come near to anyone who experiences healing and that we are emissaries of God's kingdom, present as that close encounter happens. We'll conclude that healthcare work is properly understood as gospel work.

THE LAMB AND THE KING

The New Testament expresses its good news in a variety of ways. To fully appreciate the role of healing in the gospel, we need to consider two biblical images that convey the good news: Jesus the Lamb and Jesus the King.

Jesus is "the Lamb of God, who takes away the sins of the world" (Jn 1:29). To Jesus' Jewish disciples, this phrase was an obvious reference to the sacrificial system established by the Mosaic law, in which an innocent lamb's blood was spilled to make payment for people's misdeeds. Jesus, the Lamb of God, was uniquely qualified to pay the penalty for our waywardness, once and for all, by his sacrificial death on our behalf.

The necessity of Jesus' sacrifice for us can seem odd to a modern sensibility. But think of what it's like to be alienated from someone who was previously close to you. The restoration of that relationship will be painful and will require a sacrifice of some sort—at least one of the persons involved will have to admit they were wrong, lay aside their claims, or make payment for loss. Renewal of relationship also requires the willingness of both parties, and sometimes the intervention of a third party is needed.

Human alienation from God is the same sort of problem, but the alienation is more comprehensive and profound, the gap between parties is much larger, and the solution (the shedding of blood) is more radical. Furthermore, we can't remedy it on our own. My human brokenness, my inclination to stray from God, and my tendency to fall short of his standard in my thoughts, words, and deeds separates me from him. This alienation is not easily resolved: it requires a sacrifice beyond what I can offer. Jesus chose to die on my behalf in order to remove the barriers that separate me from my Father. I participate in the reconciliation Jesus obtained for me by willingly accepting it and giving him my allegiance.

Jesus' death on the cross is the key element of this aspect of the good news. My many violations of God's standard are forgiven, once and for all, if I believe Jesus sacrificed himself on my behalf, restoring me to God. Because of his sacrifice for me, I call Jesus "Savior."

Jesus is also a king. He is the ruler of a kingdom called "the kingdom of heaven" or "the kingdom of God," which he frequently taught about. His claim to lordship over a kingdom is rooted in his role in creation: through him the world was made and is sustained, and life as we know it derives from him (Jn 1:1-4; Heb 1:2-3). With his coming to earth as a man, the kingdom of God had come near to ordinary people and circumstances in the person of Jesus himself (Lk 17:21). Jesus said that his kingdom is "not of this world," meaning it is not part of the global political order, but it is breaking into the world and setting creation right (Lk 16:16; Jn 18:36). His kingdom is demarcated not by geographical borders but by his sovereign leadership (Lk 17:20-21), and it is populated by people who identify as his citizens—a personal change so radical he called it being "born again" (Jn 3:3-5).

Jesus walked the earth as a king without comfort, recognition, or wealth. He taught that his kingdom is near, open to all, and requires a personal response of repentance. He spent his time with the marginalized, the poor, the sick, and the hungry, meeting their needs and transforming their lives—and he calls his followers to do the same (Mt 10:8; 25:44-45; Lk 6:28; 12:33-34). I walk through life as a member of his kingdom by practicing repentance, following his example, and obeying his direction.

Jesus' resurrection is the key element of this aspect of the good news. By his remarkable power, God raised Jesus from the dead, thereby negating death's power over everyone who belongs to his kingdom (Heb 2:10-18). Through his life and resurrection, King Jesus blazed a path for us. He gives us the strength to follow him and enables us to live as children of God. Because of his kingship, I call Jesus "Lord."

Jesus is both Lamb and King, our Savior and our Lord. There is nothing contradictory about these two images. In fact, they reinforce and amplify each other (Col 1:15-22). Jesus' formulation of the gospel—"The kingdom of God has come near. Repent and believe the good news"—puzzled me because I had a flattened understanding of the gospel. I knew Jesus as my Savior, but I was missing my place in his kingdom and his kingdom's impact in the here and now. Because Jesus has reconciled me with God, bringing me into his kingdom, I have the opportunity to play my part in his grand redemptive project. This fuller understanding of the good news helps explain why healing is part of Jesus' work. He is healing our brokenness as our Savior, and he is healing his creation—in part, through healthcare—as its King.

HEALING AND THE KINGDOM

When John the Baptist was in prison, he heard what Jesus was doing and wondered whether he really was the Messiah, the long-promised Savior-King of Israel. John sent messengers to Jesus, asking, "Are you the one who is to come, or should we expect someone else?" (Mt 11:3). Jesus did not answer with a simple, "Yes, I am the Messiah" or "No, I am not the Messiah." Instead he offered evidence: "Go back and report to John what you hear and see: The blind receive sight, the lame walk, those who have leprosy are cleansed, the deaf hear, the dead are raised, and the good news is proclaimed to the poor" (Mt 11:4-5). In answering this way, Jesus was referring to prophetic descriptions of the Messiah's kingdom as a place where blindness and deafness are cured, streams break forth in the desert, predators no longer kill, sadness and sorrow flee away, and God's people experience everlasting joy (Is 35:5-10). God's kingdom is a place where creation is set right again and the curses of Genesis 3 are lifted.

Healing, then, was not an arbitrary aspect of Jesus' ministry, an ancillary activity or afterthought. Healing was vital evidence of the King's presence and his kingdom's reality. Healing is also central to the future, fully realized kingdom of God on earth, described near the end of the book of Revelation: "He will wipe every tear from their eyes. There will be no more death or mourning or crying or pain, for the old order of things has passed away" (Rev 21:4). Healing is a feature of the kingdom of God across the sweep of time, from Old Testament prophecy, through Jesus' ministry, to Revelation's account of the end of our era. Healing that occurs now is part of this continuum. It is an exhibition of the kingdom's reality and an indicator of Jesus' royal presence. Healing is a sign that Jesus and his kingdom have come near.

As we saw in chapter four, all healing is a gift from God, regardless of whether that healing appears to be by miraculous or medical means. Scientific knowledge, surgical techniques, medical therapies, and our bodies' healing abilities are all part of God's common grace shown to all people. When our patients experience healing, the kingdom of God has come near to them. This is true whether or not the patient or their healthcare professional recognize it.

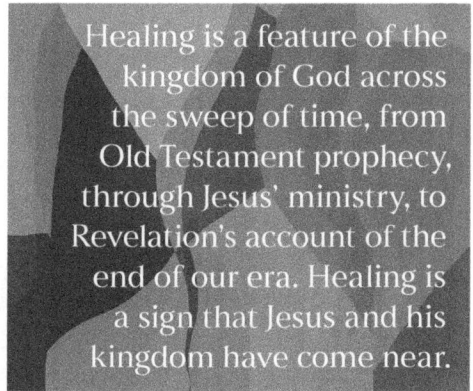

> Healing is a feature of the kingdom of God across the sweep of time, from Old Testament prophecy, through Jesus' ministry, to Revelation's account of the end of our era. Healing is a sign that Jesus and his kingdom have come near.

HEALTHCARE WORK IS GOSPEL WORK

Our patients are having close encounters with Christ's kingdom through the experience of medical care, healing, and our presence. Let's look at how we can benefit from this truth in our day-to-day work as healthcare professionals:

Recognize that God is at work in our clinics and hospitals. God has brought our patients to us, and through their medical issues he is working out his purposes in their lives. We can choose to think of our wards, clinics, offices, operating rooms, and emergency departments as outposts of the kingdom of God. The relief of symptoms and recovery from illness that we routinely facilitate and often take for granted are exhibitions of God's grace and, for the patient, a visceral and timely experience of the goodness of Jesus. We rightly take satisfaction from the role we play in that process. That's one reason why fulfillment comes when we perceive God's presence at our workplace. It's energizing to recognize that we embody his love and care in healthcare settings, using the skills and abilities he's given us to live out our purpose as his citizens.

Be an ambassador. A recent poll asked US adults, "When you consider your spiritual beliefs, what would you say you are looking for?" The top three responses were inner peace, hope, and healing.[2] Certainly people coping with illness are looking for these as well! Christ's kingdom is a place where people find peace, hope, and healing. We are ambassadors of the kingdom, representatives of Jesus, and guides to the spiritual resources many of our patients are looking for.

What does it look like to be an ambassador of the kingdom? We can be the salt of the earth by bringing a satisfying flavor to our interactions with others (Mt 5:13). We can be the light of the world by speaking out for what is true, pure, lovely, excellent, and praiseworthy (Mt 5:14). We can be the fragrance of Christ by permeating our workplaces with the pleasing presence of God's love (2 Cor 2:15).[3] People can get a glimpse of Jesus when the fruit of God's Spirit is exhibited in our lives—love, joy, peace, patience, kindness, goodness, faithfulness, gentleness, and self-control—qualities that no one objects to (Gal 5:22-23). These are often most noticeable when they are most needed, for instance, in times of stress or conflict. When we are kind to patients and coworkers, even when they don't deserve it, they have a personal experience of grace—and our kindness is often contagious.[4] When we are the ones who don't argue or complain (Phil 2:14-15) but freely

When we are the ones who don't argue or complain (Phil 2:14-15) but freely give others our time and attention (Mt 5:41-42), we are like yeast working its way all through a batch of dough (Mt 13:33), influencing our workplace for the kingdom.

give others our time and attention (Mt 5:41-42), we are like yeast working its way all through a batch of dough (Mt 13:33), influencing our workplace for the kingdom.

Point to the good news. Healing often brings with it hope, gratitude, and a sense of fresh opportunity. When we see these in our patients, it's sometimes appropriate to reflect these feelings toward God. Oftentimes we can do this by asking questions, for instance, "How has this experience affected your spirit?" or with simple comments that don't require a response: "I've been praying for you, and I'm so glad you're better." "I thank God you've done so well."

Only some of our patients will recognize that the kingdom of God has come near them. When, in the course of clinical care, we mention spirituality—for instance, by taking a spiritual history, as I did with the patient I described at the start of this chapter, or by telling our patients we've been praying for them—we've placed spirituality on the table with our patients. We have cracked open a window through which a breeze of spiritual reality can flow. For some of our patients, this will be like fresh air entering a stuffy room; for others it will be unwelcome or irrelevant. In almost all healthcare settings, we can ask about our patient's spiritual journey, we can affirm that spirituality matters, and we can open the door to spiritual renewal. Some of our patients will choose to walk through that door—to, in Jesus' words, "repent and believe the good news."

Embrace kingdom priorities. The kingdom's values are distinctive and refreshing. We align with Jesus as we champion kingdom ways of living and working. The kingdom is a community where forgiveness is experienced and passed forward (Mt 18:23-35), where all ethnicities and races are represented (Lk 13:28-30), and where the marginalized and irreligious are welcomed (Mt 9:9-13). In the kingdom the usual social pecking order— from the rich and powerful down to the poor and vulnerable—is flipped upside down (Mk 10:17-25; Mt 18:1-5). It's a place where seemingly small investments can grow large over time (Mk 4:30-32). Kingdom members treasure the kingdom more than wealth or recognition (Mt 13:44). They move toward life's messes.[5]

When we live out these values people notice:

- A student fellowship group I know brings care packages to hospitalized patients after getting approval from the ward nursing staff. The staff welcomes their visits and alerts them to certain needy patients.
- A nurse started bringing flowers to the unit where she works. She says that her coworkers are now more likely talk to her about their lives.
- Another friend apologized to his coworkers for having been irritable and cross: "I was wrong, and I'm sorry." He says it was not easy to humble himself this way—to admit how un-Christlike he'd been—but since then his behavior at work has improved and his work relationships have deepened.

All of these healthcare colleagues would tell you they have found satisfaction in being kingdom citizens at work.

We are together the body of Christ. Most of us have friends, coworkers, and patients who are also members of God's global kingdom. Like every effective organization, the kingdom is composed of smaller units—churches, fellowships, prayer groups, accountability partners—that facilitate its work. We are not lone rangers. Linking with other members of Jesus' kingdom in our workplaces can be particularly important for those of us who day after day pour ourselves into healthcare. We can help each other see the reality of the kingdom in our workplace. Find a time and place to meet with a fellow believer while you're both at work to share and pray together. Use the reflections and exercises at the end of this chapter to jump-start your conversations.

FOR REFLECTION

1. Why is the nearness of God's kingdom good news?
2. According to Matthew 4:17 and Mark 1:15, the appropriate response to the nearness of God's kingdom is repentance. Why is this so? (See chapter six.)
3. Was healing central only to Jesus' gospel or also to the gospel of his disciples? (See Lk 9:1-2; 10:8-9.)

4. How can you point to the gospel in your work context? Consider 1 Peter 3:15 and the examples in the latter half of this chapter. Is the gospel best left to chaplains, or can other healthcare workers participate?

IT'S YOUR TURN

We benefit from recognizing the kingdom of God at our workplaces, but, for many of us, it doesn't come naturally. It can be easy to miss the nearness of God's kingdom in healthcare. Here are some ways to practice seeing and being part of the kingdom this week:

1. Can you spot Jesus at work this week in your hospital or clinic, mending his creation? Keep a five-day record of the times the kingdom of God was evident to you at work. When you start, it may help to reflect back at the end of each shift or workday, or when you're taking a break, identifying these moments in retrospect. Put "kingdom spotting" on your calendar as a daily item or appointment. If you can't identify instances of God at work in your healthcare context, ask him to show them to you.

2. As ambassadors of Christ's kingdom, we stand out from the default culture we live and work in. Review the list of the fruit of the Spirit found in Galatians 5:22-23. Which of these is most lacking from your work persona? (For me, it's often patience.) In the coming week, pray daily on the way to work and while you're at work for the Spirit to produce this quality in you. If someone asks, tell them that the quality they've noticed in you is the result of God working in your life.

3. Put spirituality on the table with at least one of your patients every day this week. You don't have to have all the answers to their spiritual questions or even offer them any answers. Use context-appropriate, nonthreatening means such as taking a spiritual history, mentioning you've been praying for them, asking how their spirit is doing, or offering referral to a spiritual counselor such as a pastor or chaplain.

12

Why Jesus Went into Healthcare

ONE DAY I RECEIVED a phone call from a doctor at another hospital, asking to transfer a patient to our intensive care unit. The patient was a successful businessman who lived in an affluent suburb. He had fallen ill with a severe gastrointestinal illness, complicated by respiratory failure requiring mechanical ventilation. He was getting worse, and there was a real possibility he could die. My colleague mentioned that the patient's wife was angry. I realized that he was worried about a potential lawsuit.

Together with my ICU colleagues I accepted the patient, and he was brought to our hospital by ambulance. I was unable to converse with him, as he was on a ventilator and sedated, but his wife visited daily, and we talked. At first she asked pointed questions about her husband's treatment, which I answered as best I could. I began to understand that her expectations for the future had been shaken. As the days went by, she accepted that we were doing our best and began to tell me about her husband's drinking and about the loneliness and stress of their lives. During bedtime prayers with my young daughters, we would often pray for one of my patients, and we began to pray for this patient nightly.

The patient slowly improved. He was extubated and moved to a regular hospital ward. He started eating and walking. One afternoon I sat in his hospital room and we discussed discharge plans together. "I'm delighted by how well you're doing. My daughters and I have been praying for you, and now we can stop," I said. The patient and his wife both looked at me, alarmed. "Please don't stop!" they responded. They asked about finding a church to attend.

The satisfaction I felt caring for this man and his wife was the sort of thing I had hoped for from a healthcare career. I had the pleasure of using my professional skills to help heal a patient. I felt the fulfillment of being both competent and caring. And I was able to encourage my patient's spiritual health.

Why do people go into healthcare professions? There are many reasons. In surveys, the majority of healthcare students, doctors, and nurses indicated that helping others was a top motivation for pursuing their career.[1] One survey of medical students found that reasons clustered into two categories: professional calling and personal growth.[2] "Professional calling" included serving in a noble profession, helping others, and becoming a role model. "Personal growth" included job stability, good salary, wide career options, and prestige and respect in society.

Jesus spent time healing people. Why did he go into healthcare? We've already identified programmatic reasons: he came to heal whole persons, bodies included, reversing the curses of Genesis 3. He is a king, and his kingdom is a place where people are rescued and healing happens. These reasons are true, but they don't explain why Jesus chose to heal people one at a time. Surely he could have banished disease from whole swaths of the population at once. But instead, his healing acts were personal encounters, much as ours are with our patients. Why did he choose to heal individuals one by one? In the four Gospels there are over thirty accounts of Jesus' healing work, and often Jesus' motivations for healing are stated or implied. Among the many factors that moved Jesus to heal individuals, two consistently appear: his compassion for hurting people and the opportunity healing provided to demonstrate who he was.

These two motivations shaped his approach to healing. Compassion and demonstration can also shape our approach to our patients and the meaning we derive from our work.

COMPASSION

Compassion is a caring concern for others that leads us to help them. It's different from empathy, which is the ability to share in another person's feelings.[3] Too much empathy can lead us to overidentify with our patient's distress and degrade our ability to take care of them effectively. Compassion requires us to understand our patient's feelings but not to take them onto ourselves. Compassion encompasses kindness, interest, readiness to get involved, and the desire to meet another's need.

Compassion is rooted in love—not romantic love or friendship love but what New Testament writers called *agapē*: goodwill and benevolence toward another person.[4] Compassion goes beyond sympathy. It's love in action, motivated by the desire for another person's good. Of the many possible motivations for helping others, compassion is the one driven by love, expecting nothing in return.

As the following examples show, Jesus often healed out of compassion:

Jesus went through all the towns and villages, teaching in their synagogues, proclaiming the good news of the kingdom and healing every disease and sickness. When he saw the crowds, he had compassion on them, because they were harassed and helpless, like sheep without a shepherd. (Mt 9:35-36)

"What do you want me to do for you?" [Jesus] asked.

"Lord," they answered, "we want our sight."

Jesus had compassion on them and touched their eyes. Immediately they received their sight and followed him. (Mt 20:32-34)

As he approached the town gate, a dead person was being carried out—the only son of his mother, and she was a widow. And a large crowd from the town was with her. When the Lord saw her, his heart went out to her and he said, "Don't cry."

Then he went up and touched the bier they were carrying him on, and the bearers stood still. He said, "Young man, I say to you, get up!" The dead man sat up and began to talk, and Jesus gave him back to his mother. (Lk 7:12-15)

In each of these instances, Jesus responds to serious and sometimes desperate human need by both caring *about* people and caring *for* them. Compassion mattered in Jesus' ministry, and it matters today because sick people are whole persons. Their physical plight often leaves their souls and spirits thirsty for compassion.

Recent randomized controlled trials of compassionate patient care have shown decreased peri-operative depression and anxiety, improvements in stress and symptom perception in persons living with inflammatory bowel disease, and better control of eating disorders with compassion-based interventions.[5] Compassion instills efficacy into patient encounters because it is medicine for hurting souls and spirits.

Compassion makes a measurable difference in patient care. Between 2005 and 2008, "conditions of appalling care were able to flourish" at a hospital serving the people of Staffordshire, England. Following a public outcry, government inquiries found a lack of basic elements of care, a focus on financial metrics rather than clinical outcomes, treatment of patients and families with "callous indifference," and high mortality rates at the hospital. The inquiries recommended changing the hospital culture by requiring staff to commit to "putting the patient first" and "a compassionate and caring service."[6] A policy titled "Compassion in Care" was put in place, promoting values of care, communication, and compassion, and outlining strategies for change.[7] By 2016, follow-up reports documented improvements in the hospital culture and patient outcomes.[8]

In chapter eight I mentioned that compassion fatigue is common in healthcare professionals today. It is the weariness that builds as our reservoir of goodwill and benevolence toward others dries up. I easily run out of compassion, especially when I'm tired and overworked. At such times I can still manage to treat my patients according to the standard of care, even though my heart isn't in it. This might lead me to conclude that compassion is optional in healthcare. But both the clinical data already mentioned and the spiritual realities of healthcare say otherwise. Paul writes:

> If I speak in the tongues of men or of angels, but do not have love, I am only a resounding gong or a clanging cymbal. If I have the gift of prophecy and

can fathom all mysteries and all knowledge, and if I have a faith that can move mountains, but do not have love, I am nothing. If I give all I possess to the poor and give over my body to hardship that I may boast, but do not have love, I gain nothing. (1 Cor 13:1-3)

This passage is often read at weddings, but it is more relevant to our work. If Paul had been writing specifically to healthcare professionals, I can imagine him saying something like, "If I cure thousands of patients but do not have love, I am only a sophisticated algorithm. If my professional skills are unparalleled but I do not have love, I am nothing special. If I work long hours and make a good living but do not have love, I have gained nothing at the end of the day."

These verses teach us that love brings meaning to human interactions. They highlight that when we care about others, we gain, meaning we benefit in ways we otherwise would not. Research demonstrates that when we help others out of compassion—not simply because it's our job to help—our own well-being improves.[9] Our compassion benefits our patients, and it also brings us fulfillment. That's why, when we lack compassion, our work dwindles in significance and our work-related satisfaction fades.

What does it look like when a Christian healthcare professional loves their patients? The rest of 1 Corinthians 13 tells us: we are patient, kind, not proud, not dishonoring, not self-seeking, not easily angered. We always protect, always trust, always hope, always persevere. We are gentle and considerate. We pay attention to our patients and take time to answer their questions. We give them the benefit of the doubt. We look out for their best interest. None of these features of compassion are dependent on clinical outcomes, nor are they primarily emotions we feel. They are behaviors that spring from our caring concern for people. They are choices we make, expressions of compassion.

How Patients Sense Compassion

Patients sense compassion when we greet them warmly, get to know them, listen carefully to them, show that we like them, give them the benefit of the doubt, and treat them with respect. Compassionate communication is unhurried and attentive, and avoids interrupting the other person. It presents information sensitively and clearly, checks for understanding, and can be confrontational when necessary. It makes effective use of silence, giving patients room to gather their thoughts and respond to our questions. In many cultures, compassion can be communicated nonverbally by making eye contact, smiling, nodding to indicate understanding, warming our hands before touching our patients, and adopting an open body posture as we talk with them.[a] As a patient, I've experienced compassion when my nurse brought me an extra blanket or offered me a hot drink. These were physical encouragements I needed at the time. Children, nervous in their pediatrician's office, are on the receiving end of compassion when their caregiver tells them a joke or tosses them a stuffed animal.

[a]Shane Sinclair, Jill M. Norris, Shelagh J. McConnell, Harvey M. Chochinov, Thomas F. Hack, Neil A. Hagen, Susan McClement, and Shelley Raffin Bouchal, "Compassion: A Scoping Review of the Healthcare Literature," *BMC Palliative Care* 15, no. 6 (2016): 1-16, https://bmcpalliatcare.biomedcentral.com/articles/10.1186/s12904-016-0080-0.

It can be difficult to have caring concern for our patients. Sometimes it has to do with the patient: they may be unkempt, unpleasant, noncompliant, unappreciative, or lacking insight. They may have a seemingly unending list of health complaints or present us with a complex, challenging clinical situation. Other times it has to do with us: we may be weary, overworked, emotionally fatigued, hardened by patient care, and unable to make the personal commitment to our patients that compassion requires. Sometimes it has to do with the systems we work in: they may encourage an assembly-line approach to patients and have expectations, incentives, and values that discourage compassion and lead to professional burnout.

The compassion we have for others builds as the compassion we experience ourselves increases.[10] How do we get on the receiving end of compassion, recharging our batteries for clinical care? Equitable working conditions, sympathetic supervisors, help with stress and moral injury when needed, and sufficient time away from work all create room for us to refill our stores of compassion. Work-hour limits are particularly important.[11] "Self-compassion" training, which promotes acceptance of ourselves rather than self-criticism, can improve psychological health. Spiritual practices are an important means by which we receive compassion and benefit from it. One recent study showed that a compassion intervention based on religious instruction was superior to a secular intervention.[12]

Paul writes that God is "the Father of compassion and the God of all comfort, who comforts us in all our troubles, so that we can comfort those in any trouble with the comfort we ourselves receive from God" (2 Cor 1:3-4). For Christians, God is our primary source of compassion, and the compassion we receive from him enables us to show compassion to others. We are conduits, not generators, of compassion. Personal devotional time and a rhythm of regular participation in a community of faith—at a church, study group, or fellowship—can give us opportunities to experience God's comfort and renew our compassion. We can also benefit from God's caring concern when, instead of being self-sufficient on the job, we turn to him in the middle of our workflow. As we humble ourselves before him—conceding that we need his help—his Spirit comforts and strengthens us. "The Spirit helps us in our weakness" (Rom 8:26).[13] When we sense God walking with us (Ps 23:4) while we're at work, and take a moment to decompress into the reality of his goodness and love, his Spirit restores our compassion and equips us to fulfill our purpose.

> For Christians, God is our primary source of compassion, and the compassion we receive from him enables us to show compassion to others. We are conduits, not generators, of compassion.

God uses our compassion in the lives of patients who are on a journey toward him. Only occasionally, though, might we learn what happens after they leave our care. "I hear you were Ms. Hammersmith's doctor in the hospital," a nonmedical friend of mine said to me one day. "Is that so?" I responded, mentally reviewing her case. She had been admitted with an infection, which had responded well to standard treatment. She had been one of many patients I had cared for during a busy month, and I had no idea she and my friend were coworkers. "She told me you were kind to her, and something you said gave her the sense you're a Christian," he continued. "I invited her to my Bible study group. What did you say to her, anyway?" With confidentiality issues in mind, I said to my friend, "I really can't comment." I mentally reviewed her case again. I could think of nothing unusual about our interactions. Jesus, using an agricultural analogy, said that some of us sow seed, and others reap a harvest. In healthcare we often have the opportunity to sow seeds of compassion.

DEMONSTRATION

A second overarching factor that motivated Jesus to heal was the opportunity healing provided to demonstrate his true nature. Jesus was the long-anticipated Lamb of God who came to take on our plight, sacrificing himself for us. Healing showed how effectively Jesus the Lamb could shoulder our burdens: "When evening came, many who were demon-possessed were brought to him, and he drove out the spirits with a word and healed all the sick. This was to fulfill what was spoken through the prophet Isaiah: 'He took up our infirmities and bore our diseases'" (Mt 8:16-17). Jesus takes our weaknesses and illnesses on himself. He carries them, suffering on our behalf. His nature is demonstrated to our patients when they experience healing. When we bring our workplace fatigue to him, his power is demonstrated as he takes it onto himself, lightening our load.

Jesus is also a king, the Creator embodied in his own creation, with kingly power over all of nature, including human health. Jesus often chose to heal in ways that emphasized his authority over creation:

> He said to the paralyzed man, "Son, your sins are forgiven."
>
> Now some teachers of the law were sitting there, thinking to themselves, "Why does this fellow talk like that? He's blaspheming! Who can forgive sins but God alone?"
>
> Immediately Jesus knew in his spirit that this was what they were thinking in their hearts, and he said to them, "Why are you thinking these things? Which is easier: to say to this paralyzed man, 'Your sins are forgiven,' or to say, 'Get up, take your mat and walk'? But I want you to know that the Son of Man has authority on earth to forgive sins." So he said to the man, "I tell you, get up, take your mat and go home." He got up, took his mat and walked out in full view of them all. (Mk 2:5-12)

Jesus healed this paralyzed man in a way that challenged those present by drawing attention to his divine nature. His healing work demonstrated Jesus the Lamb and Christ the King taking on our infirmities and restoring whole persons, reversing the brokenness of our world and our lives.

Jesus combined compassion and demonstration in his healing work. For instance, John 11 tells the story of Lazarus's illness, death, and resurrection. Lazarus and his sisters Mary and Martha were friends of Jesus, but when he heard Lazarus was sick, Jesus delayed two days before traveling to see him. By the time Jesus arrives Lazarus was dead and buried, and a wake was in progress. Jesus tells Martha that he is more powerful than death: "I am the resurrection and the life. The one who believes in me will live, even though they die" (Jn 11:25). When Jesus sees Mary crying, his love for Lazarus surfaces: he is "deeply moved in spirit and troubled" (Jn 11:33) and weeps himself. Jesus then raises Lazarus from the dead. Compassion and demonstration, love and power, are intertwined throughout this account.

If Jesus healed as a demonstration, can we too heal in ways that demonstrate who he is? In the last chapter we saw that Jesus and his kingdom come near to people who experience healing, but sometimes they're oblivious to that spiritual reality. Often demonstration starts with compassion: our caring concern communicates God's love to our patients. Demonstration links our compassion—and the healing our patients experience—with the reality of Jesus' presence and love.

> Demonstration links our compassion—and the healing our patients experience—with the reality of Jesus' presence and love.

Pointing to Jesus' role in our patients' healing doesn't involve preaching a sermon. Often, in the context of a busy medical or nursing practice, it requires only a single sentence or phrase: "I've been praying for you," or "Someone upstairs has been looking out for you," or "I thank God you're better," or "I think God has done something special for you." These expressions do not require a response from our patients, and they're not meant to challenge our patients' faith background. They are simple reflections of the spiritual reality we perceive.

We have opportunities to demonstrate Jesus to our patients at a time when he is already at work in their lives. How we do so will depend on our diagnosis of their spiritual state. When we demonstrate truths about Jesus, we gain: we align ourselves with God in real time, and we experience his presence in the middle of our workflow.

COMPASSION AND DEMONSTRATION
IN OUR DAILY PRACTICE

I'm best for my patients, and also benefit the most myself, when I care for my patients with compassion and demonstration. That's because, at the end of the day, "the only thing that counts is faith expressing itself through love" (Gal 5:6). How, in practical terms, can we make compassion and demonstration integral to our healthcare practices?

Be compassionate. Helping and compassion are different. Helping is what you do; compassion is the way you do it. Helping requires a set of medical skills, and compassion requires a loving approach. The sidebar earlier in this chapter describes some of the behaviors that demonstrate compassion to our patients; these are generalities that will vary somewhat between cultures. When you pray for yourself, ask for help being compassionate with your patients. Our most difficult patients may be the ones who most need our caring concern.

Compassion is key to satisfaction in a healthcare career. Sometimes it comes naturally. But what can we do when it doesn't? The first step is to recognize that our heart is not in our work. Sadly, I sometimes realize this only when others let me know I've been uncaring. At other times I recognize my own lack of compassion when, in retrospect, I regret an interaction or simply when my work stops being satisfying. The next step is diagnostic: Does my lack of compassion indicate overwork, or physical, mental, or moral fatigue? Is it a sign that I am out of touch with God and spiritually unhealthy myself? Is it the result of an inequitable workplace culture that needs a systemic solution? It can help to discuss the situation with a trusted friend or mentor.

If the issue, at least in part, lies with us, we can recover or strengthen compassion as we attend to our own physical and spiritual health—something that can be hard to do in the middle of an all-consuming career but that is necessary if we're to be more than "resounding gongs or clanging cymbals." Taking care of our bodies (as discussed in chapter two), carving out regular time to nurture our Christian identity, and experiencing God's caring concern for us while we're at work are key to finding fulfillment in the work God has put in our hands.

At times I try to act compassionately even though I don't feel it. Compassionate body language and words are part of my professional persona, and acting compassionately can jump-start the care I feel for my patient by reminding me of my calling in real time. But in the long run, an awareness of God's presence best sustains my caring concern for others, because God is the source of compassion.

Demonstrate Jesus. We are, first and foremost, children of God and members of his kingdom. In almost every healthcare context there are means to make faith visible in winsome and uncontroversial ways, and opportunities to point to the power and love of Jesus in response to the questions people ask. For instance:

- Symbols such as a cross on a necklace, or a Bible in your consultation room, are forms of demonstration. A friend who works in an emergency department wears a cross lapel pin. He says that patients notice and sometimes ask him to pray. Other times the emergency room staff asks him to stand in when a chaplain is not available.

- Conversations provide opportunities to share who we are. A patient asked a physical therapist I know about her plans for the weekend, and the therapist mentioned she would be going to church. The following week, at the beginning of their next therapy session, the patient said, "I want you to know I was diagnosed with cancer a couple of weeks ago. I'm scared. You're one of the few people I've told." The patient began to cry. My friend responded, "That must be so difficult. Thank you for sharing." "Would you pray for me?" the patient asked. "Yes, I'd love to," my friend said. She prayed with her patient right there in the physical therapy session.

- Taking a spiritual history (as discussed in chapter three), offering biblical wisdom in response to patient needs (chapters four and six), praying for or with patients (the next chapter), and giving God credit for healing (chapter four) can all point patients to Jesus.

We have the opportunity to speak about Jesus when we're asked to share spiritual perspectives in the context of a trusted relationship. Oftentimes it's wise to start by telling about our own experience or the anonymized experience of our patients. How do we begin to describe our experience of Jesus with simple, nontheological language to patients and coworkers when appropriate? Some examples are shown in the sidebar.

Expressing Our Experience of Jesus

"Faith has made all the difference for me in difficult times."

"Prayer is important to me. It brings me comfort and peace."

"After my dad's death, his spirit felt very close to me, and I'm convinced his spirit lives on. It's one of many ways spirituality is important to me."

"Thanks to Jesus, I feel free from the mistakes of my past."

"In tough times we all need peace and hope. For me, Jesus is the best source."

"Some of my patients say that God gives them the strength and hope they need in times like this."

"Our patients need our compassion, but it's hard to sustain that day after day. On my best days I know that God is here and that he loves me. He gives me what I need for my patients."

"Like everyone, I want to earn a living wage. But I think our work is about more than money. It's about sharing God's love and helping people experience the goodness of healing."

Having shared some of our experience, we can keep the dialogue going by asking a question such as, "What do you think about that?" or "Is faith important to you?" or "Have you ever felt God nudging you?" After relating some of our own spiritual history, we often have the freedom to ask about the other person's spirituality, even in contexts where religion is infrequently discussed.

Improvise. Healthcare in resource-rich settings rarely involves improvisation. We rightly aim to practice according to standards and algorithms. But neither compassion nor demonstration is algorithmic. In the Gospel accounts, Jesus rarely heals the same way twice. He perceives the unique needs and circumstances of hurting people and responds in ways that best fit the situation. "Love is improvisation" because our patients are unique individuals.[14] One size does not fit all. Compassion focusses us on our patients' needs, not our own compulsions, and gives us the freedom to act and speak in ways that best encourage each patient. Demonstration also best flows from the desire to understand each patient's spiritual state and discern how to encourage their spiritual health rather than raising barriers in their lives to spirituality. Sometimes our patients need compassionate action from us, not words; at other times they need a listening ear, human touch, encouraging words, a Scripture verse, or prayer. As you consider how to demonstrate Jesus, be motivated by love, not guilt. We become better at improvisation—and discover new forms of professional fulfillment—as we tune our hearts to the Holy Spirit's promptings in our workplace.

FOR REFLECTION

1. When do you struggle to show compassion to your patients? How do you best show compassion to your patients? Recall that compassion is a disposition of the heart—a caring concern for others—and is expressed through a set of behaviors. Discuss with a colleague.

2. How do you demonstrate Jesus to your patients in contextually appropriate ways? Review the examples mentioned in this chapter and exchange ideas with friends.

3. Do you find it hard to love (*agapē*) your patients? To what extent is this due to the nature of your patients, the system you work in, or your own physical and spiritual health? What can you do to recover or strengthen a Christlike approach?

IT'S YOUR TURN

Compassion flows through us to others. Our sense of purpose and satisfaction grows as we increasingly know ourselves as channels of God's comfort. It's your turn to work on this during the coming week:

1. Remember that compassion is caring concern for others—it's not primarily about sharing in their feelings. Identify factors that are blunting your caring concern for patients. Are you fatigued and overworked? Are you feeling distant from God? Do the expectations and values of the system you work in discourage compassionate caregiving? If you perceive systems issues, make time to discuss them with an interested mentor or supervisor.

2. Psalm 23 describes God's caring concern for us. Pray it at the start of each workday, either before you leave home, while you're on the bus, or after you park your car in the lot. Say the verses one by one to God in prayer, pausing after each verse to tell God what it means to you. Print out the psalm and put it where you'll see it at work— maybe next to your keyboard or inside your locker or lunch bag.

3. As you move through your workday, notice whether you have a heart of caring concern for the patients and coworkers you're with. When you're running low on compassion, take a moment to relax into your faith. Thank the Spirit that he is with you, tell him you can't do it without him, and ask him for comfort.

4. Demonstrate Jesus to your patients. In many healthcare contexts this involves physical cues or simple statements that don't require a response. Use the sort of practical methods and words described in this chapter to demonstrate Jesus to others. These methods not only communicate to our patients; they align us with Jesus at work.

13

How Much Faith Is Enough?

A WOMAN WITH SEVERE COLITIS was admitted to my hospital service. She had been diagnosed one month previously, and since then her diarrhea and rectal bleeding had worsened, despite treatment. She now had anemia, abdominal pain, and fever. Her x-rays did not show a toxic megacolon that might require urgent surgical removal of her colon, and we opted for intravenous medical treatment, knowing that surgery might become necessary.

I asked whether faith was part of her life, and she said yes. She became tearful when I asked whether her faith had been important to her during her illness. "When I got sick I gave money to my church, and the pastor prayed for me to be healed, but it didn't help," she said. "My pastor says it's because I don't have enough faith."

Faith is indispensable to the practice of modern medicine. Without faith in us and biomedical science, patients would not come to us for care or agree to undergo uncomfortable procedures or take potentially toxic medications. And the broadly recognized power of placebos is evidence of the impact faith has on healing within the biomedical paradigm. The placebo effect accounts for up to 50 percent of the therapeutic benefit of medications and surgery in clinical practice.[1]

In the Gospels a person's openness to the possibility of healing—and willingness to ask for healing—often frame the context in which Jesus heals. In this chapter we'll look at the degree of faith Jesus required from the people he healed. We'll see that tentative faith, mixed with doubt, was sufficient—and that the healing process sometimes led people to faith. We'll apply this to our work by exploring how asking Jesus for healing today—through prayer—can help our patients experience the benefits of faith, even if they are skeptics. Praying for and with patients in a nuanced, respectful, and contextually appropriate manner can encourage our patients' spiritual health and align us with our purpose as we work.

ATTITUDE MATTERS

On one occasion, Jesus returned to his hometown in the course of his itinerant ministry. He was not well received there:

> When the Sabbath came, he began to teach in the synagogue, and many who heard him were amazed.
>
> "Where did this man get these things?" they asked. "What's this wisdom that has been given him? What are these remarkable miracles he is performing? Isn't this the carpenter? Isn't this Mary's son and the brother of James, Joseph, Judas and Simon? Aren't his sisters here with us?" And they took offense at him.
>
> Jesus said to them, "A prophet is not without honor except in his own town, among his relatives and in his own home." He could not do any miracles there, except lay his hands on a few sick people and heal them. He was amazed at their lack of faith. (Mk 6:2-6)

People were amazed by Jesus wherever he went, but the amazement of people in his hometown differed. They knew him and his family from childhood, and when he returned home, preaching with confidence and having a newfound reputation as a miracle worker, they were wary and took offense at him. Perhaps they suspected a scam, or dismissed the possibility that the boy they had known was now a powerful healer. Maybe they were indignant, thinking that he seemed to have surpassed them: Who did he think he was, anyway? It appears that only a few sick people were receptive enough or desperate enough to come to him for healing.

Contrast the attitude of his hometown neighbors with the attitude of a man who came to Jesus because his child was sick:

There was a certain royal official whose son lay sick at Capernaum. When this man heard that Jesus had arrived in Galilee from Judea, he went to him and begged him to come and heal his son, who was close to death.

"Unless you people see signs and wonders," Jesus told him, "you will never believe."

The royal official said, "Sir, come down before my child dies."

"Go," Jesus replied, "your son will live."

The man took Jesus at his word and departed. While he was still on the way, his servants met him with the news that his boy was living. When he inquired as to the time when his son got better, they said to him, "Yesterday, at one in the afternoon, the fever left him."

Then the father realized that this was the exact time at which Jesus had said to him, "Your son will live." So he and his whole household believed. (Jn 4:46-53)

In this case, a royal official comes to Jesus because of his son's illness. Although he is an important person in society, he humbles himself and begs Jesus to heal his son. Jesus' initial response implies that the official is a skeptic—but he ducks Jesus' challenge about faith and pleads again for his son. When Jesus tells him that his son will live, the official takes Jesus at his word, suggesting that faith has taken tentative root in his heart. It's only later, after he confirms the details of his son's healing, that the royal official is said to believe in Jesus.

Why are there divergent outcomes in these two instances? In both examples people are skeptical of Jesus. But in the second passage, the royal official in his desperation sought Jesus out and humbled himself before him, honoring him rather than taking offense, respectfully asking Jesus to heal his son. Healing followed, and belief came even later.

We can conclude from these examples that, when it came to healing, a person's attitude toward Jesus mattered. They had to be receptive to the possibility that Jesus could heal. They had to be willing to humbly ask him for help. But they may nevertheless have been unsure about Jesus. They may not yet have given him their allegiance. Jesus did not require wholehearted belief from those he healed. Consider the case of an epileptic boy who was possessed by a demon:

When the spirit saw Jesus, it immediately threw the boy into a convulsion. He fell to the ground and rolled around, foaming at the mouth.

Jesus asked the boy's father, "How long has he been like this?"

"From childhood," he answered. "It has often thrown him into fire or water to kill him. But if you can do anything, take pity on us and help us."

"'If you can'?" said Jesus. "Everything is possible for one who believes."

Immediately the boy's father exclaimed, "I do believe; help me overcome my unbelief!"

When Jesus saw that a crowd was running to the scene, he rebuked the impure spirit. "You deaf and mute spirit," he said, "I command you, come out of him and never enter him again."

The spirit shrieked, convulsed him violently and came out. The boy looked so much like a corpse that many said, "He's dead." But Jesus took him by the hand and lifted him to his feet, and he stood up. (Mk 9:20-27)

This father has brought his son to Jesus, seeking healing. His skepticism is revealed by the way he asks for help: "If you can do anything. . . ." His doubt is understandable, because Jesus' disciples had already failed to help the boy, as related earlier in the text. Jesus, after taking a medical history, raises the issue of faith. In response to Jesus' challenge, the father claims to believe but also admits unbelief. His faith is wavering and tentative. Yet Jesus nevertheless exorcises a demon and restores the boy's health.[2]

Willingness to pursue the possibility of healing is necessary for biomedical healing to occur: unless sick people seek medical care, they can't benefit from medical treatment. The same holds true for healing Jesus offers. "You do not have because you do not ask God" (Jas 4:2). When Jesus tells people, "Your faith has healed you" (Mk 5:34; 10:52; cf. Eph 2:8-9), he is affirming that their willingness to ask for healing was a prerequisite for the healing he performed. I once cared for a seminary student with a chronic illness that had not responded well to initial treatment. He had been sent for a second opinion. As we discussed therapeutic alternatives, I asked him whether he had prayed about his illness. "No," he responded. "That's okay for my congregation, but I wouldn't pray for healing for myself." "Any port in a storm!" I responded, hoping to encourage him to try prayer.

Some of our patients have a similar view of Jesus as the royal official or the father of the epileptic boy. They may be unsure about faith, sitting on the fence, undecided. Or perhaps they haven't given their spirituality much thought before, but illness has caused them to ask spiritual questions. Or, if they're spiritually curious, they may be disinterested in traditional religion but desire spiritual experiences and resources. In any of these cases, our patients may now admit the possibility that God is present and that he can hear and heal, and they may be willing to humble themselves and try asking God for healing. This attitude seems to be acceptable to Jesus. He will work with a sliver of tentative faith. Elsewhere Jesus uses the example of a mustard seed of faith as sufficient for effective prayer (Mt 17:20). The mustard seed is a tiny seed that grows into a large plant, and like all seeds it is full of dormant potential. "It is the object of your faith, not the quality or purity of your faith, that saves you."[3]

> Jesus will work with a sliver of tentative faith.

Faith often exists in the presence of doubt. We believe not because we have no doubts but because faith best explains our world and our experience of God. For some doubting patients, prayer is a means of taking faith for a test drive. It may be their first attempt (or their first attempt in a long time) to adopt the posture and behavior of a believer. Jesus hears their prayer, and he may choose to heal them as he did the royal official's child and the father's epileptic son. When we pray a simple lament with our patients, we're demonstrating how they can turn to God.

Willingness to humbly ask for help is all Jesus requires of us. A corollary of this conclusion is that lack of healing, despite prayer for healing, isn't due to insufficient faith. Our doubts and reservations don't stop Jesus. Patients who have prayed for but do not experience bodily healing may struggle with feelings of inadequacy or experience a crisis of faith. Yet the issue is not the quality or quantity of their faith. We may have the opportunity to reframe their understanding, as discussed in chapters two, four, six, and nine. To the woman I described at the start of this chapter, I said, "I'm a Christian too, and I'm impressed that you've turned to God for help with this illness. Many people don't. You know, the Bible says that a tiny amount of faith is enough. I think God loves you and hears you and is here with you. Let's stay in touch with him as we walk through this together."

A CALLOUSED HEART

While some of our patients are like the royal official or the father of the epileptic boy, others are like the citizens of Jesus' hometown: disinterested in spirituality, or perhaps wounded by prior encounters with religion, and not about to pray for help. About such people, God says, "For this people's heart has become calloused; they hardly hear with their ears, and they have closed their eyes. Otherwise they might see with their eyes, hear with their ears, understand with their hearts and turn, and I would heal them" (Acts 28:26-27).

A calloused heart prevents healing. This is true with regard to modern medicine: persons who are skeptical of biomedical science and choose not to seek medical care, or who reject medical advice, often miss opportunities for healing. A person whose heart is calloused toward God may similarly miss out on the physical, emotional, or spiritual healing he offers. For some people their intellectual doubts, past experiences of judgment or hypocrisy from Christians, or anger toward God have created calluses of the heart that prevent them from dipping their toes into faith, even when they're sick. The best medicine in these situations may be to love our patients and pray for them in the hope that the power of God and the experience of compassion will soften their hearts.

ENCOURAGING OUR PATIENTS' SPIRITUAL HEALTH

Here are practical ways to apply these insights to your practice and discover the satisfaction that comes from modeling and encouraging spiritual health in healthcare settings:

Meet patients where they are. When you take a spiritual history, remember that Jesus worked with people's wavering and uncertain faith. Your patients who long ago let go of religious routines, are nursing hurts inflicted by the church, or are curious about angels, demons, and seances may all have embers of faith waiting to be fanned into flame, to their own benefit.

Don't dismiss what might seem to you a flimsy spirituality. Help them take their next step toward (or back toward) God. How you do that will vary with the person—but in healthcare contexts, it rarely involves a sermon. We are used to giving people answers to their questions about health, but many of our skeptical or spiritually curious patients are less interested in spiritual answers than in guidance that helps them explore spirituality themselves.[4] Sometimes simply asking questions and hearing about their spiritual journey is the place to start. We can ask, "Have you ever felt that God was pursuing you?" or "Tell me about a person whose spiritual life you really admired."[5] Suggesting that they daily find things to thank God for, or read Psalm 23 or the Gospel of Mark, or modeling for them how to pray, or referring them to an effective religious counselor may be appropriate. Remember to suggest small, practical steps they can take. List spiritual diagnoses such as "spiritual distress" or "readiness for enhanced religiosity," and follow up on them as you do with other diagnoses.

Offer to pray with your patients. The people in the gospel stories we've considered talked to Jesus face to face. For us, prayer is our means of asking Jesus for healing. It often seems easiest to pray with patients who express a strong religious faith and are used to prayer. But prayer also gives our patients who are spiritually curious a chance to try wading into the ocean of belief. Our prayer with them may be a skeptic's first venture in faith. Prayer is one way of walking with our patients a few steps along the pathway toward spiritual health. How much faith does Jesus require of them? Only enough to humbly ask for help.

> Prayer is one way of walking with our patients a few steps along the pathway toward spiritual health.

Can prayer be therapeutic? A meta-analysis of ten randomized controlled trials of intercessory prayer in acute care settings, including over seven thousand patients, found no statistically significant effect of prayer on physical health outcomes, although there was a nonsignificant trend toward lower mortality among patients receiving prayer.[6] To maintain blinding, these studies used prayer offered by persons who were at a distance from the sick individual and had never met or talked with the sick person they were praying for. The patients were not told to pray themselves, and they did not know whether prayer was being offered on their behalf. This, of course, is not how people asked Jesus for healing, or how we typically practice prayer.

More recent randomized studies have shown that religious and spiritual interventions augment patient well-being and quality of life, beneficially impact some physiological parameters, and improve symptoms of depression and anxiety in patients with various clinical problems, including cancer, cardiovascular disease, chronic pain, and mental illness.[7] In these studies, patients themselves participated in spiritual interventions. This research suggests that our patients can benefit when they pursue spiritual health through activities such as prayer.

Prayer makes God a member of a patient's care team. Al Weir tells the story of a Christian surgeon he calls Jason, whose patient

> presented with an advanced, but not hopeless malignancy. She had once been Jewish but gave up her faith in God when her husband died young. From the beginning, Jason encouraged her to understand that God was in charge. When he asked if she would like to invite God into her illness, she immediately agreed, so he prayed with her. Jason and the patient and God had been visibly working together with an initial great response to therapy. Now it looks as if the cancer has returned and will someday take her life. Rather than letting God slip out of the picture and assume He had failed his patient, Jason continues to pray with her. She does not yet embrace God, but she is pondering his possible presence. This week, in fact, she was passing a church and decided to enter. She told Jason that the priest provided for her a moment of peace. "You see," Jason told her, "God loves you and has shown Himself for your comfort."[8]

How can we discern which patients to offer prayer to? Sometimes patients allude to faith or express religious concerns, alerting us to their interest in prayer. More often, spiritual history-taking reveals which patients are not open to prayer and which patients may be receptive. Here is how one group of oncology researchers put it:

> Many patients with advanced cancer view prayer with their clinician as appropriate, but appropriateness is case-specific and depends on multiple factors. Taking a spiritual history equips practitioners to navigate religion

and spirituality on a case-by-case basis, recognizing that although the role of prayer should always remain voluntary, practitioners hold a central role as facilitators of spiritual care in the setting of advanced illness.[9]

Remember that Jesus' love for the people he encountered shaped his approach to them and that our insights into our patients similarly guide our interactions.

If you choose to offer prayer to your patient, how can you raise the subject? It's important to offer in such a way that they're free to decline without feeling they have undermined their healthcare or their relationship with you. For instance, a surgeon I know says as he is wrapping up pre-operative visits, "One more thing: I always offer to pray with my patients. If you're interested in that, let me know." Offer prayer in a way that focuses on the patient's need for healing, not your need to pray with them. I don't say, "I'm going to pray with you now," or ask, "Is it OK if I pray for you?" I much prefer the question a colleague of mine asks her patients: "Would it help if I prayed with you?" You don't want your patient to feel like an object being prayed over but instead like a (often silent) participant in your prayer. If they decline your offer, reassure them that's OK with you.

When you do pray with a patient, consider using the lament form of prayer on their behalf (chapter nine). The elements of a lament demonstrate a posture toward God that promotes healing, and are highly relevant to patients' needs. These elements can be expressed simply and briefly using the TREAT acronym: tell God your patient's need, remember God's love and faithfulness, ask boldly for help, trust in God. For example: "God, we know you're here with us now. Ms. Petrov is suffering [or unwell, or in pain]. I know that you love her, have watched over her life, and have brought her here for treatment today. Please bring healing to her through [the treatment we've planned, or the operation we're doing]. We trust you." Avoid preaching during your prayer, or using theological terms, or asserting denominationally divisive ideas. For some patients it may be appropriate to ask whether they want to pray too.

Some patients may be alarmed that we're offering prayer, taking this as a sign that we don't think we can help them, that we expect a bad outcome, or that we lack confidence in our professional skills. Consider approaches that forestall these conclusions. For instance, you could mention that you always pray for your patients or that you often offer to pray together with them. Include in your prayer thanksgiving for the capable care team God has provided.

Prayer has the potential to set our patients up for disappointment. Avoid implying that prayer will cause healing to occur or "claiming" healing in prayer. The decision to heal is God's, not ours. Express confidence in the goodness of God, not in the outcome. Remember that faith may be therapeutic for our patients in multiple ways: the possibility of direct miraculous healing, thankfulness for God's common grace gift of medical treatment, healing of the soul and spirit, freedom from fear, and God's gift of peace that passes understanding.

FOR REFLECTION

1. Do you think that a patient's faith in their caregiver affects their decisions about treatment and their response to treatment? Why or why not?

2. What is the minimum evidence of faith that Jesus requires for healing?

3. Does lack of healing equate to lack of faith? How would you respond to a patient or visiting family member who expresses this viewpoint?

4. When might you offer prayer to a patient who has doubts about faith? How would you go about it?

5. Might prayer for healing set our patients up for disappointment and disillusionment? How can this pitfall be avoided?

IT'S YOUR TURN

1. If you've never prayed with a patient before, the idea may seem overwhelming. Start by praying for your patients, not with them. Offer a brief, silent prayer—including elements of a TREAT prayer—before or after each patient encounter. As this becomes habitual, you may find that opportunities to pray with your patients come into view.

2. Ask God to prompt you to offer prayer to a patient this week. Based
on their spiritual history, and when you feel the Spirit nudging you,
you might start by saying that you often pray for patients and then
ask, "Would it help if I prayed with you?" If the patient says no,
accept their disinterest gracefully—reassure them that that's fine. If
they say yes, pray a brief lament on their behalf, telling God their
situation, mentioning God's love and faithfulness, asking boldly for
healing, and affirming trust in God. Don't limit offers of prayer to
patients who you know share your particular religious affiliation.

Conclusion

WHEN I GOT TO work yesterday, I found out that my patient load had doubled. A colleague had called in sick. Someone had to fill in for them, and I was the only available resource—so I had twice as many patients as usual.

As you might imagine, I was cross. Was my colleague really that sick? How could they have saddled me with so much extra work? Why doesn't our system take these sorts of unexpected absences more fully into account? There should be a better backup plan! As I started seeing patients, I noticed that our entire team was on edge. Everyone was annoyed by the circumstances.

Our third patient made me pause. She seemed anxious. I wondered whether the vibe that I and our whole team were feeling had somehow spread to our patients. God's presence flickered into my awareness. I realized that the tone of the day needed to change—my tone especially. I slowed down and asked the patient to tell me about herself. I asked what concerns were on her mind. I put a hand on her shoulder. These simple, momentary actions realigned me with my purpose. I remembered that God was her Father, my Father, and Father of all of us working together that day. Something tight inside of me unwound.

My fourth patient was a priest. After the usual clinical interaction, I asked him whether he wanted to pray for us. He was abashed—we were in a secular healthcare setting—and he declined. A nurse who knows that I sometimes pray with patients heard all of this and couldn't quite suppress a laugh.

After that the day went smoothly. All of us found small ways to recognize the worth of our patients: asking about their lives, apologizing for delays, sharing some encouraging words. We worked hard, but the irritation was gone. It was replaced by satisfaction in the work, for me and for the rest of my team, I believe. In the early afternoon additional help arrived, and we finished just an hour later than usual. I went home surprisingly content.

The spiritual dimension of healthcare practice brings us satisfaction. It's there in almost every clinical encounter, waiting to be recognized. Sometimes it's a placid stream, supporting us like water floats a boat. Other times it's a cresting wave that we can choose to surf. When we welcome it, we see our patients and their health in three dimensions. We relax into our faith, and we experience the comfort that the Spirit brings us. We know ourselves to be instruments of God's favor. We align with our purpose: to heal creation, reflecting God's love and care into people's lives.

As you discover God's presence at the point of care, remember that clinics and hospitals are outposts of his kingdom, places where he is working, and that he often chooses to work through us. Tune yourself to his presence through the personal practice of repentance, worship, and prayer. Look for opportunities to encourage the spirits of the people you work with and care for. I'm praying that God's Spirit will continue to nudge both me and you while we're at work, reminding us that he is close, giving us insight into our patients, restoring our compassion, and renewing our joy in healthcare!

Notes

INTRODUCTION

[1]Throughout this book I often use the words *medicine* and *medical* to refer broadly to all sorts of healthcare work, and those of us who regularly interact with patients, including (but not limited to) clinical assistants, dentists, dental hygienists, dietitians, emergency medical technicians, nurses, nurse practitioners, pharmacists, phlebotomists, physicians, physician assistants, registered nurses, surgeons, and occupational, physical, and speech therapists.

[2]There is currently pushback against the concept of a calling to a healthcare career. Calling has been depicted as an institutional tool used to justify long work hours, systemic inequities, and unsatisfactory work conditions for healthcare professionals. See Lisa Rosenbaum, "On Calling—from Privileged Professionals to Cogs of Capitalism?," *New England Journal of Medicine* 390, no. 5 (2024): 471-75, http://doi.org/10.1056/NEJMms2308226. This is an important critique; an equitable work environment is a necessary (though not sufficient) basis for thriving at work, and the concept of a calling should not be used to maintain unjust or unhealthy working conditions. *Calling* has become a secular term thanks to "workism," a replacement for faith that portrays work as "the centerpiece of one's identity and life purpose." See Derek Thompson, "Workism Is Making Americans Miserable," *The Atlantic*, February 24, 2019, www.theatlantic.com/ideas/archive/2019/02/religion-workism-making-americans-miserable/583441/. I have in mind an older concept of calling: God's offer to us of roles in his redemptive work in the world. For Christians, calling occurs in the context of an identity that is rooted in and relating to Christ. It's within this type of calling that work-related meaning and satisfaction blossom, without work defining who we are.

CHAPTER 1: BEING HUMAN

[1]Names and other details have been changed or withheld in all of the clinical stories I tell in this book to protect the privacy of my patients and colleagues.

[2]Randy Cohen, Chirag Bavishi, and Alan Rozanski, "Purpose in Life and Its Relationship to All-Cause Mortality and Cardiovascular Events: A Meta-Analysis," *Psychosomatic Medicine* 78 (2016): 122-33, doi: 10.1097/PSY.0000000000000274; Ian D. Boreham and Nicola S. Schutte, "The Relationship Between Purpose in Life and Depression and Anxiety: A Meta-analysis," *Journal of Clinical Psychology* 79 (2023): 2736-67, doi: 10.1002/jclp.23576.

[3]Some scholars refer to God's instruction to be fruitful and multiply as the cultural mandate, meaning that we create and pass on a legacy that reflects the image of God into creation. In this view, we fulfill our creaturely mandate not only by having children but by shaping, investing in, and discipling future generations. See Greg Beale, "What Is the Relationship Between the Cultural Mandate and the Great Commission?," *Gospel Coalition*, May 19, 2017, YouTube video, 2:05, www.youtube.com/watch?v=CGJZeSFyzs0.

[4]Carmen Joy Imes, *Being God's Image: Why Creation Still Matters* (Downers Grove, IL: IVP Academic, 2023), chap. 2.

[5]James I. Packer, "Reflected Glory," *Christianity Today* (December 2003), www.christianitytoday.com/2003/12/reflected-glory/; C. S. Lewis, *The Weight of Glory* (San Francisco: HarperOne, 2001), 45-46; Imes, *Being God's Image*, chap. 1.

[6]Timothy J. Keller, *Every Good Endeavor: Connecting Your Work to God's Work* (New York: Penguin Books, 2014), 48.

[7]Nicholas T. Wright, "Mind, Spirit, Soul and Body: All for One and One for All: Reflections on Paul's Anthropology in His Complex Contexts" (lecture, Society of Christian Philosophers, Fordham University, March 18, 2011), https://ntwrightpage.com/2016/07/12/mind-spirit-soul-and-body.

[8]See Col 3:23-24 and Andy Crouch, *Playing God: Redeeming the Gift of Power* (Downers Grove, IL: InterVarsity Press, 2013), chap. 1; Wright, "Mind, Spirit, Soul and Body."

[9]Francis A. Schaeffer, *Genesis in Space and Time* (Downers Grove, IL: InterVarsity Press, 1972), 46-47. For more on the concept of spirit, see chapter two of this book.

[10]See Eccles 3:21; Gen 6:17; 7:15, where *ruakh* (a Hebrew word commonly translated "spirit") is used in reference to animals.

[11]Francis A. Schaeffer, *Escape from Reason* (Downers Grove, IL: InterVarsity Press, 1968), chap. 4.

[12]The parallelism between Gen 5:1-2 and Gen 5:3 is a form of intentional repetition that implies a direct relationship between concepts. The idea that all humankind has a family relationship with God is also found in Eph 3:14-15; Rom 8:29.

[13]Timothy Keller, "The Centrality of the Gospel" (sermon preached at Redeemer Presbyterian Church, New York, November 2, 1997).

[14]Ursula Meidert, Godela Dönnges, Thomas Bucher, Frank Wieber, and Andreas Gerber-Grote, "Unconscious Bias among Health Professionals: A Scoping Review," *International Journal of Environmental Research and Public Health* 20 (2023): 6569, doi: 10.3390/ijerph20166569.

[15]Philosopher Peter Singer proposes that our value is rooted in our abilities or capacities and that an incapacitated person may have less value than an animal. See Singer, *Animal Liberation Now* (New York: Diversion Books, 2023). The Christian understanding of human value is rooted in our nature, not our capacities.

[16]Daniela C. Augustine, "Image, Spirit and Theosis: Imaging God in an Image-Distorted World," in *The Image of God in an Image-Driven Age*, ed. Beth F. Jones and Jeffrey Barbeau (Downers Grove, IL: IVP Academic 2016), 173-88.

[17]Anne E. K. Roberts and Katrina Bannigan, "Dimensions of Personal Meaning from Engagement in Occupations: A Metasynthesis," *Canadian Journal of Occupational Therapy* 85 (2018): 386-96, doi: 10.1177/0008417418820358.

[18]The analogy of a broken or fractured mirror for the "image of God" is found in the writings of the nineteenth-century politician and theologian Abraham Kuyper (*To Be Near Unto God*, chapter 44, https://ccel.org/ccel/kuyper/near/near.xlv.html). For a recent application, see Mark Matlock. *Faith for the Curious: How an Era of Spiritual Openness Shapes the Way We Live and Helps Others Follow Jesus* (Grand Rapids, MI: Baker Books, 2024), chap. 1.

[19]A number of related quotations expressing this concept have been attributed to Mother Teresa. For instance, "I know I am touching the living body of Christ in the broken bodies of the hungry and the suffering. Each one of them is Jesus in disguise." "Quotes from Mother Teresa," *Vision, Values and Aims* (blog), accessed December 27, 2024, https://blogs.glowscotland.org.uk/ed/turnbullvva/quotes-from-mother-teresa/.

[20]Al Weir, personal communication.

[21]For more on how to develop the skills of a supercommunicator and how these skills can lead to better clinical decisions, see Charles Duhigg, *Supercommunicators: How to Unlock the Secret Language of Connection* (New York: Random House, 2024).

[22]Dustin A. Demming, quoted in "Q&A: Oncologist's Colorectal Cancer Diagnosis 'Changed the Way I Interact with Patients,'" Healio, August 11, 2023, https://www.healio .com/news/gastroenterology/20230810/qa-oncologists-colorectal-cancer-diagnosis -changed-the-way-i-interact-with-patients.

[23]Duhigg, *Supercommunicators*, 42-49.

[24]Vivek Murthy, "Health Worker Burnout," United States Department of Health and Human Services, May 25, 2022, https://www.hhs.gov/surgeongeneral/reports-and -publications/health-worker-burnout/index.html.

CHAPTER 2: BODY

[1]For instance, see Mt 22:37-40; 25:31-46; Lk 4:18-19; 10:25-37; Jas 2:14-17. A full investigation of the theological debate between prioritism, which emphasizes preaching the gospel, and holism, which teaches that sharing the gospel and addressing the physical needs of others are both important for Christians, is beyond the scope of this book. Some claim that our responsibility to help others with their physical needs is limited to our own faith community, but certain texts suggest otherwise: the good Samaritan was not a Jew

but helped a Jew, and it's unlikely that the "strangers" referred to in Matthew 25 were part of the local house church. Jesus combined word and deed in his own outreach (Lk 24:19), and he urged us to love our enemies (Mt 5:43-48). We are told to bless those who persecute us, often by responding to their physical needs (Rom 12:14-21).

2Basilides, a Gnostic philosopher, writes, "Salvation belongs to the soul alone, for the body is by nature subject to corruption." As quoted by Irenaeus, *Against Heresies* 1.24.5, trans. Alexander Roberts and William Rambaut, in *Ante-Nicene Fathers*, vol. 1, ed. Alexander Roberts, James Donaldson, and A. Cleveland Coxe (Buffalo, NY: Christian Literature, 1885), www.newadvent.org/fathers/0103124.htm. For more on Gnosticism's influence on our modern view of the body, see Nicholas T. Wright, "Mind, Spirit, Soul and Body: All for One and One for All: Reflections on Paul's Anthropology in His Complex Contexts" (lecture, Society of Christian Philosophers, Fordham University, March 18, 2011), https://ntwrightpage.com/2016/07/12/mind-spirit-soul-and-body; Gregg Allison, *Embodied: Living as Whole People in a Fractured World* (Grand Rapids, MI: Baker Books, 2021), 11-20.

3John Wilkinson, "The Body in the Old Testament," *Evangelical Quarterly* 63, no. 3 (1991): 195-210.

4There are several religious theories about the origin of souls. Some world religions—but not Christianity—believe that souls preexist bodies and are joined to them at conception. Christians differ on whether God creates individual souls at the time of physical conception and places them in the developing fetus (the "creation theory") or whether our souls are inherited from our parents, like our bodies (the "Traducian theory"). See Gregory Brown, "Origin of the Soul," Bible.org, 2021, https://bible.org/seriespage/5-origin-soul; Wright, "Mind, Spirit, Soul and Body."

5"Towb," in *A Hebrew and English Lexicon of the Old Testament*, by Francis Brown, S. R. Driver, and Charles A. Briggs (Peabody, MA: Hendrickson Academic, 1994), www.biblestudytools.com/lexicons/hebrew/nas/towb-2.html.

6Tim Mackie, "What Does It Mean to Be Evil?," *Bible Project* (podcast), October 16, 2023, https://bibleproject.com/podcast/what-does-it-mean-be-evil/.

7Wright, "Mind, Spirit, Soul and Body."

8Scripture refers to circumcision of the heart (Deut 30:6; Rom 2:29), and Col 2:9-12 depicts baptism as a form of circumcision of "your whole self" (Col 2:11).

9If bodies are essential to our being, how can we exist without them in the interval between death and resurrection? The Bible tells us that we will immediately be with Jesus when we die, even though our mortal bodies are dead and decomposing (2 Cor 5:8; Lk 23:43)—but Paul suggests there is something unwelcome about this intermediate state (2 Cor 5:3-4). Gregg Allison writes of life in the intermediate state between death and resurrection: "We as disembodied people continue to live with Christ in heaven . . . [but] because the proper state of human existence is embodiment, as disembodied people in heaven, we will long for and anticipate the resurrection of our body. Then, and only then, will our salvation be complete" (*Embodied*, 20).

Physical things, our bodies included, exist in space and time. God, on the other hand, is spirit and exists outside as well as inside time. When we die, we will immediately be with God, outside time. We will be plunged back into time at the resurrection and continue in time thereafter. If this conjecture is true, then in our own experience of life after death there will be no time during which we are without a body—even though, to observers on earth, our bodies will have decomposed and centuries may pass between our death and resurrection. Medicine provides a partial analogy: when awaking from general anesthesia patients often have no sense of time having passed, even though their operation took hours. To be outside time is to be in a changeless, static state, but we were made to respond to change, enjoy change, and instigate change ourselves. We were made for space and time. When we re-enter space and time as resurrected bodies, our salvation will be complete, and we will thrive as active citizens of Christ's new heaven and new earth.

How (if at all) will I be a different person when I am resurrected? The Bible tells us our resurrected bodies will be permanent and impervious to the ravages of time and disease. If our current bodies are like tents, temporary and contingent, our resurrected bodies will be like houses. If our current bodies are like seeds, destined to fall into the ground and die, our resurrected bodies will be like the plants that sprout from seeds (2 Cor 5:1-5; 1 Cor 15:35-44). These biblical metaphors show us that resurrected bodies will be more substantial, more real than our bodies are now. And, it's not only our bodies that will be transformed at the resurrection. Using the image of a seed, Paul writes, "It is sown a natural body, it is raised a spiritual body. . . . And just as we have borne the image of the earthly man, so shall we bear the image of the heavenly man" (1 Cor 15:44, 49). The Greek words here translated as "natural" and "spiritual" are adjectives that derive from the nouns *psychē* and *pneuma* and that are often translated "soul" and "spirit," the topics of the next chapter. N. T. Wright points out that these adjectival forms "describe not the material out of which things are made but the power or energy that animates them." Wright, *Surprised by Hope* (San Francisco: HarperOne, 2008), chap. 10. Our "natural bodies" are animated by our *psychē*: the life force that is our emotion, ambition, desires, and personality. Our resurrected selves will be imperishable bodies animated by *pneuma*, our spirit communing with the life-giving spirit of Jesus. When animated by *pneuma*, we will be attuned to and in sync with Jesus, united with him in a new way.

[10]A proper discussion of the biblical approach to disability is beyond the scope of this book. Both scholars and disabled persons have increasingly highlighted that disability, at least in some forms, does not need correction and is not inconsistent with health. Our value as human beings derives from our being made in the image of God, not from our abilities or capacities. See, for instance, Bethany McKinney Fox, *Disability and the Way of Jesus: Holistic Healing in the Gospels and the Church* (Downers Grove, IL: IVP Academic, 2019).

[11]The Greek word often translated "flesh" is *sarx*, which can refer to the body in a positive sense (e.g., Jn 1:14; Eph 5:31). However, *sarx* often has negative connotations in the Pauline

epistles, where it can refer not to the physical body but to our wayward human nature, opposed to God and prone to sin ("sarx," in Brown, Driver, and Briggs, *Hebrew and English Lexicon*, www.biblestudytools.com/lexicons/greek/nas/sarx.html). When this meaning is intended, *sarx* is sometimes contrasted with the body itself or the "members" (limbs and organs) of our bodies. For instance, in Rom 7:5 Paul writes, "While we were living in the flesh [*sarki*], our sinful passions . . . were at work in our members [*melesin hēmōn*] to bear fruit for death" (ESV). Our passions express themselves bodily. Sadly, this verse describes some of our patients, who suffer medically because of their poor choices or the wrongdoing of others. Paul is not, however, characterizing our bodies as evil. Similarly, he elsewhere writes, "Do not let sin reign in your mortal body so that you obey its desires, and do not present your members to sin as instruments to be used for unrighteousness, but present . . . your members to God as instruments to be used for righteousness" (Rom 6:12-13 NET). Here the parts of our bodies are called "instruments" or tools, which can serve either good or evil purposes. Consider surgical instruments such as scalpels or scissors, beautifully designed tools with the potential for good or evil, which are used by a surgeon to accomplish something good. So too our bodies are here depicted as key components of our commitment to either righteous or unrighteous living.

John Vervaeke offers "self-destruction and self-deception" as a modern explication of the ancient term *sin*. See, e.g., "Making Sense of the Meaning Crisis | John Vervaeke," Planet: Critical, October 20, 2022, YouTube video, 1:09, www.youtube.com/watch?v=qilGa6Al5BY. This description highlights one aspect of sin: when we fall short of what's best or opt to disobey God, our behavior runs counter to our own ultimate self-interest.

[12]Christoffer Grundmann, "Christ as Physician: The Ancient *Christus medicus* Trope and Christian Medical Missions as Imitation of Christ," *Christian Journal for Global Health* 5, no. 3 (2018): 3, http://doi.org/10.15566/cjgh.v5i3.236.

[13]Allison, *Embodied*, 20. N. T. Wright expresses the same idea: "Ultimate salvation is not in heaven but in the resurrection into the combined reality of the new heaven and the new earth" ("Mind, Spirit, Soul and Body").

[14]E.g., Lk 4:31-44. The Greek word translated "preach" in Lk 4:44 can also be translated "evangelize," incorporating both word and deed in a summary of Jesus' ministry approach. Miraculous healing certainly validated Jesus' words, but this was not the only purpose healing served in his ministry: on some occasions he healed without preaching.

[15]Matthew Loftus, "When an Abortion Is Pro-life," *New York Times*, May 20, 2022, https://www .nytimes.com/2022/05/20/opinion/abortion-doctor-pro-life.html?searchResultPosition=1.

[16]Zhiyu Dong et al., "Negative Effects of Endoscopists' Fatigue on Colonoscopy Quality on 34,022 Screening Colonoscopies," *Journal of Gastrointestinal and Liver Disease* 30, no. 3 (2021): 358-65, http://doi.org/10.15403/jgld-3687.

[17]Tiina Ritvanen, Veikko Louhevaara, Pertri Helin, Toivo Halonen, and Osmo Hänninen, "Psychophysiological Stress in High School Teachers," *Stress* 24, no. 6 (2021): 998-1007, https://pubmed.ncbi.nlm.nih.gov/14587539/; Günther Neumayr and Peter Lechleitner,

"Effects of a One-Week Vacation with Various Activity Programs on Cardiovascular Parameters," *Journal of Sports Medicine and Physical Fitness* 59, no. 2 (2019): 335-39, https://pubmed.ncbi.nlm.nih.gov/29498252/; Elaine D. Eaker, Joan Pinsky, and William P. Castelli, "Myocardial Infarction and Coronary Death Among Women: Psychosocial Predictors from a 20-Year Follow-Up of Women in the Framingham Study," *American Journal of Epidemiology* 135, no. 8 (1982): 854-64, https://pubmed.ncbi.nlm.nih.gov /1585898/.

[18]Qi Miao et al., "Three Cases of Karoshi Without the Typical Pathomorphological Features of Cardiovascular/Cerebrovascular Disease," *American Journal of Forensic Medicine and Pathology* 41, no. 4 (2020): 305-8, http://doi.org/10.1097/PAF.0000000000000600.

CHAPTER 3: SOUL AND SPIRIT

[1]For a discussion of the various scholarly approaches to soul and spirit, see J. K. Chamblin, "Psychology," in *Dictionary of Paul and His Letters*, ed. Gerald F. Hawthorne, Ralph P. Martin, and Daniel G. Reid (Downers Grove, IL: InterVarsity Press, 1993), 765-75.

[2]Nicholas T. Wright, "Mind, Spirit, Soul and Body: All for One and One for All: Reflections on Paul's Anthropology in His Complex Contexts" (lecture, Society of Christian Philosophers, Fordham University, March 18, 2011), https://ntwrightpage.com/2016/07/12 /mind-spirit-soul-and-body.

[3]For instance, 1 Thessalonians 5:23; 1 Corinthians 15:44. See chap. 2 n9 for a discussion of this passage.

[4]Wright, "Mind, Spirit, Soul and Body."

[5]Based on a word study of the Hebrew *nephesh* and the Greek *psychē*. These words for "soul" typically refer to living biological beings or the characteristics that are typical of or essential for life. Particularly in the New Testament, the psyche is not depicted as the locus of our spirituality.

[6]Some authors prefer the word *mind* to the word *soul*. These are not identical terms, and they could both be included in a description of our nonanatomical selves. In 1 Thessalonians 5:23 Paul refers to people as body, soul, and spirit, thereby giving us a "multifaceted description of the whole" of a human being (Wright, "Mind, Spirit, Soul and Body"). I've chosen to emphasize the word *soul* rather than *mind* because the Greek word *psychē* can encompass more than our awareness and cognition, and because consciousness may best be thought of as a product of body, soul, and spirit functioning together.

[7]Based on a word study of the Hebrew *ruakh* and the Greek *pneuma*. Unlike *soul*, these words for "spirit" may refer not only to biological beings but also to God, angels, or demons. When applied to people, these words may refer to the commonality through which God relates to and equips us.

[8]Jesse L. Preston and Faith Shin, "Spiritual Experiences Evoke Awe Through the Small Self in Both Religious and Non-religious Individuals," *Journal of Experimental Social Psychology* 70 (2017): 212-21, https://doi.org/10.1016/j.jesp.2016.11.006.

[9]The Old Testament describes mediums who can communicate with the spirits of dead people but also warns us not to engage in this activity (1 Sam 28:3-20; Lev 19:31). The Jewish leaders of Jesus' day believed that communication with other spirits was possible (Acts 23:9).

[10]1 Samuel describes the close friendship of David and Jonathan: "The soul of Jonathan was knit to the soul of David, and Jonathan loved him as his own soul" (1 Sam 18:1). Similarly, Moses speaks of friends who are "as your own soul" (Deut 13:6). Spirituality, a personal and relational attribute, may in part explain our capacity to form and maintain close bonds with other souls.

[11]In Romans 12:1, the Greek word *logikēn* has been variously translated "spiritual" and "reasonable." God's Spirit within Christians, communing with our spirits, directs our behavior by means of a spiritual logic (Jason Polk, personal communication).

[12]Humans have recognized a spiritual plane of existence for millennia, and most people affirm spiritual reality today. This implies that sensitivity to spirituality confers an evolutionary advantage, and data supporting this idea is referenced later in this chapter. In his book *Signals of Transcendence: Listening to the Promptings of Life* (Downers Grove, IL: InterVarsity Press, 2023), Os Guinness points out that the possibility of an evolutionary explanation for our appreciation of love, evil, and other spiritual realities doesn't negate their existence but instead may point to our species' evolving ability to perceive a real, immaterial element of our universe.

[13]What happens when we die? See chap. 2 n9.

[14]See David Guzik's commentary on 1 Kings 19: "1 Kings 19—God Encourages Discouraged Elijah," Enduring Word, 2024, https://enduringword.com/bible-commentary/1-kings-19/.

[15]Bessel van der Kolk, *The Body Keeps the Score: Brain, Mind, and Body in the Healing of Trauma* (New York: Penguin Books, 2015).

[16]Peter Payne, Peter A. Levine, and Mardi A. Crane-Godreau, "Somatic Experiencing: Using Interoception and Proprioception as Core Elements of Trauma Therapy," *Frontiers in Psychology* 6 (February 2015), http://doi.org/10.3389/fpsyg.2015.00093.

[17]Shangyi Bao, Mengyuan Qiao, Yutong Lu, and Yulan Jiang, "Neuroimaging Mechanism of Cognitive Behavioral Therapy in Pain Management," *Pain Research and Management* (2022): 6266619, http://doi.org/10.1155/2022/6266619.

[18]Portions of this section are adapted from the Saline Process Witness Training Trainer's Manual, version 1.4. Used with permission of IHS Global. For more information about Saline Process, visit https://ihsglobal.org/.

[19]Yoichi Chida, Andrew Steptoe, and Lynda H. Powell, "Religiosity/Spirituality and Mortality: A Systematic Quantitative Review," *Psychotherapy and Psychosomatics* 78, no. 2 (2009): 81-90, https://doi.org/10.1159/000190791.

[20]Ellen Idler, John Blevins, Mimi Kiser, and Carol Hogue, "Religion, a Social Determinant of Mortality? A 10-Year Follow-Up of the Health and Retirement Study," *PLoS ONE* 12, no. 12 (December 2017): e0189134, https://doi.org/10.1371/journal.pone.0189134.

[21]Shanshan Li, Meir J. Stampfer, David R. Williams, and Tyler J. VanderWeele, "Association of Religious Service Attendance with Mortality Among Women," *JAMA Internal Medicine* 176, no. 6 (2016): 777-85, http://doi.org/10.1001/jamainternmed.2016.1615.

[22]Adapted from the Saline Process Witness Training Trainer's Manual, version 1.4.

[23]Harold G. Koenig, "Religion, Spirituality, and Health: The Research and Clinical Implications," *International Scholar Research Notes Psychiatry* (December 2012): 278730, http://doi.org/10.5402/2012/278730.

[24]Francis A. Schaeffer, *Escape from Reason* (Downers Grove, IL: InterVarsity Press, 1968), chaps. 2-3.

[25]This paragraph is adapted from the Saline Process Witness Training Trainer's Manual, version 1.4.

[26]Kenneth I. Pargament, Harold G. Koenig, Nalini Tarakeshwar, and June Hahn, "Religious Struggle as a Predictor of Mortality Among Medically Ill Elderly Patients: A Two-Year Longitudinal Study," *Archives of Internal Medicine* 161, no. 15 (2001): 1881-85, http://doi.org/10.1001/archinte.161.15.1881; George Fitchett, Patricia E. Murphy, Jo Kim, James L. Gibbons, Jacqueline R. Cameron, and Judy A. Davis, "Religious Struggle: Prevalence, Correlates and Mental Health Risks in Diabetic, Congestive Heart Failure, and Oncology Patients," *International Journal of Psychiatry & Medicine* 34, no. 2 (2004): 179-96, http://doi.org/10.2190/UCJ9-DP4M-9C0X-835M.

[27]George Fitchett, Urs Winter-Pfändler, and Kenneth I. Pargament, "Struggles with the Divine in Swiss Patients Visited by Chaplains," *Journal of Health Psychology* 19, no. 8 (2014): 966-76, http://doi.org/10.1177/1359105313482167.

[28]Pargament et al., "Religious Struggle."

[29]Hisham Abu-Raya, Kenneth I. Pargament, Neal Krause, and Gail Ironson, "Robust Links Between Religious/Spiritual Struggles, Psychological Distress, and Well-Being in a National Sample of American Adults," *American Journal of Orthopsychiatry* 85, no. 6 (2015): 565-75, http://doi.org/10.1037/ort0000084.

[30]Xiaoxiao Wang and Chunli Song, "The Impact of Gratitude Interventions on Patients with Cardiovascular Disease: A Systematic Review," *Frontiers in Psychology* 21, no. 14 (2023): 1243598, http://doi.org/10.3389/fpsyg.2023.1243598; Geyze Diniz, Ligia Korkes, Luca Schiliró Triastão, Rosangela Pelegrini, Patrícia Lacerda Bellodi, and Wanderly Marques Bernardo, "The Effects of Gratitude Interventions: A Systemic Review and Meta-analysis," *Einstein (Sao Paulo)* (August 2023): eRW0371, https://pubmed.ncbi.nlm.nih.gov/37585888/; Michelle J. Pearce, Harold G. Koenig, Clive J. Robins, Bruce Nelson, Sally F. Shaw, Harvey J. Cohen, and Michael B. King, "Religiously Integrated Cognitive Behavioral Therapy: A New Method of Treatment for Major Depression in Patients with Chronic Medical Illness," *Psychotherapy (Chicago)* 52, no. 1 (2015): 56-66, http://doi.org/10.1037/a0036448; Marianna de Abreu Costa and Alexander Moreira-Almeida, "Religion-Adapted Cognitive Behavioral Therapy: A Review and Description of Techniques," *Journal of Religion and Health* 61, no. 1 (2022): https://pubmed.ncbi.nlm.nih.gov/34518980/.

[31]Diana L. Swihart, Siva Naga S. Yarrarapu, and Romaine L. Martin, "Cultural Religious Competence in Clinical Practice," *StatPearls* (July 2023), https://pubmed.ncbi.nlm.nih. gov/29630268/; Eve Rittenberg, "Trust, Faith and COVID," *New England Journal of Medicine* 385, no. 27 (2021): 2504-5, http://doi.org/10.1056/NEJMp2114695.

[32]Giancarlo Lucchetti, Rodrigo M. Bassi, and Alessandra L. Granero Lucchetti, "Taking Spiritual History in Clinical Practice: A Systematic Review of Instruments," *Explore (New York)* 9, no. 3 (2013): 159-70, http://doi.org/10.1016/j.explore.2013.02.004; Kristen L. Mauk and Mary E. Hobus, *Nursing as Ministry* (Burlington, MA: Jones and Bartlett Learning, 2021), chaps. 6, 9.

[33]Hannah Waite, "The Nones: Who Are They and What Do They Believe?," *Theos, London* (2022), https://www.theosthinktank.co.uk/research/2022/10/31/the-nones-who-are-they -and-what-do-they-believe.

[34]Mark Matlock, *Faith for the Curious: How an Era of Spiritual Openness Shapes the Way We Live and Helps Others Follow Jesus* (Grand Rapids, MI: Baker Books, 2024), chap. 2.

[35]Matlock, *Faith for the Curious*, chaps. 2–3.

[36]For a discussion of spiritual history-taking in nursing practice, see Mauk and Hobus, *Nursing as Ministry*, chap. 6.

[37]Kamalini Kumar, RN, PhD, personal communication. This anecdote illustrates what Dame Cicely Saunders terms "total pain," understanding that pain has psychological, emotional, social, and spiritual components. See Anita Mehta and Lisa S. Chan, "Understanding the Concept of 'Total Pain': A Prerequisite for Pain Control," *Journal of Hospice and Palliative Nursing* 10, no. 1 (2008): 26-32.

[38]Resources that give further guidance on spiritual history-taking and will help in mastering this skill include "Webinar: Dr Walt Larimore—Using a Spiritual History to Uncover Religious Struggle," ICMDA, February 3, 2023, YouTube, 53:01, www.youtube.com /watch?v=NVrU8OC2gdc&list=PLny32oCmvmF8JSWo-VpwvDV18bNE4gVVg &index=91; "Webinar: Dr Walt Larimore—Spiritual History in Clinical Practice," ICMDA, October 28, 2022, YouTube, 56:35, www.youtube.com/watch?v=FMhwZs7Qo 2Y&list=PLny32oCmvmF8JSWo-VpwvDV18bNE4gVVg&index=104; and Christian Medical and Dental Association's 2022 booklet "The Value in Taking a Spiritual History, and How to Do It."

CHAPTER 4: HEALTH AND HEALING

[1]This paragraph is adapted from the Saline Process Witness Training Trainer's Manual, version 1.4.

[2]"Survey Finds Significant Gaps in Doctor-Patient Conversations," Samueli Integrative Health Programs, October 11, 2018, www.prnewswire.com/news-releases/survey-finds -significant-gaps-in-doctor-patient-conversations-300729777.html.

[3]The WHO states that a positive vision of health "integrates physical, mental, psychological, emotional, spiritual and social well-being." "Achieving Well-being: A Global Framework," 2023, page 1, https://iris.who.int/handle/10665/376200

[4]Stan Haegert, "5-11 Virtual Missionary Support Group Video One," Christian Medical and Dental Association, 3:46, https://cmda.org/center-for-advancing-healthcare-missions/cahm-511-groups/.

[5]Roghayeh Khabiri, Leila Jahangiry, Mehdi Abbasian, Fatollah Majidi, Mahdieh Abbasalizad Farhangi, Homayoun Sadeghi-bazargani, and Koen Ponnet, "Spiritually Based Interventions for High Blood Pressure: A Systematic Review and Meta-analysis," *Journal of Religion and Health* 63 (April 2024), https://pubmed.ncbi.nlm.nih.gov/38565834/; Shashank S. Sinha, Ajay K. Jain, Sanjay Tyagi, S. K. Gupta, and Aarti S. Mahajan, "Effect of 6 Months of Meditation on Blood Sugar, Glycosylated Hemoglobin, and Insulin Levels in Patients with Coronary Artery Disease," *International Journal of Yoga* 11, no. 2 (2018): 122-28, http://doi.org/10.4103/ijoy.IJOY_30_17; Havva Sert, Merve Gulbahar Eren, Aylin Meşe Tunç, Kübra Üçgül, and Ayşe Çevirme, "Effectiveness of Spiritual and Religious Interventions in Patients with Cardiovascular Diseases: A Systematic Review and Meta-analysis of Randomized Controlled Trials," *Health Psychology* (September 2024), http://doi.org/10.1037/hea0001415.

[6]Julianne Holt-Lunstad, "Why Social Relationships Are Important for Physical Health: A Systems Approach to Understanding and Modifying Risk and Protection," *Annual Review of Psychology*, 69 (2018): 437-58, doi: 10.1146/annurev-psych-122216-011902.

[7]Liubov Louba Ben-Noun, "Figs—the Earliest Known Ancient Drug for Cutaneous Anthrax," *Annals of Pharmacotherapy* 37, no. 2 (2003): 297-300, https://pubmed.ncbi.nlm.nih.gov/12549964/.

[8]"We treat, Jesus heals" is the motto of Tenwek Hospital in Bomet, Kenya.

[9]Timothy J. Keller, *Every Good Endeavor: Connecting Your Work to God's Work* (New York: Penguin Books, 2014), chap. 10.

[10]Glenn R. Fox, Jonas Kaplan, Hanna Damasio, and Antonio Damasio, "Neural Correlates of Gratitude," *Frontiers in Psychology* 30, no. 6 (2015): 1491, http://doi.org/10.3389/fpsyg.2015.01491; Geyze Diniz, Ligia Korkes, Luca Schiliró Triastão, Rosangela Pelegrini, Patrícia Lacerda Bellodi, and Wanderly Marques Bernardo, "The Effects of Gratitude Interventions: A Systemic Review and Meta-analysis," *Einstein (Sao Paulo)* (August 2023): eRW0371, http://doi.org/10.31744/einstein_journal/2023RW0371; Ying Chen, Olivia I. Okereke, Eric S. Kim, Henning Tiemeier, Laura D. Kubzansky, and Tyler J. VanderWeele, "Gratitude and Mortality Among Older US Female Nurses," *JAMA Psychiatry* 81, no. 10 (2024): 1030-38, http://doi.org/10.1001/jamapsychiatry.2024.1687.

[11]Joshua Brown and Joel Wong, "How Gratitude Changes You and Your Brain," Greater Good, June 6, 2017, https://greatergood.berkeley.edu/article/item/how_gratitude_changes_you_and_your_brain.

[12]Xia Chen, Fang-fang Zhao, Li-xiang Zhang, Shan-bing Hou, and Ting-ting Wang, "Chain Mediating Effect of Gratitude and Meaning in Life Between Nurses' Psychological Response and Emergency Capability: A Multicenter Cross-Sectional Study," *BMC Nursing* 23, no. 1 (2024): 659, https://pubmed.ncbi.nlm.nih.gov/39285272/.

CHAPTER 5: "WHY ME?"

[1]Francis Schaeffer, *Genesis in Space and Time* (Downers Grove, IL: InterVarsity Press, 1972), 92-100.

[2]The Bible Project, "Khata/Sin," March 15, 2018, https://bibleproject.com/explore/video /khata-sin/#fn-2.

[3]Mark Matlock, *Faith for the Curious: How an Era of Spiritual Openness Shapes the Way We Live and Helps Others Follow Jesus* (Grand Rapids, MI: Baker Books, 2024), chap. 3.

[4]Donald Guthrie and J. A. Motyer, *The New Bible Commentary, Revised* (Downers Grove, IL: InterVarsity Press, 1970), 1066.

[5]Do people suffer for their parents' sins? "Passages in the Pentateuch state that God will punish offspring for the sins of their forebearers up until the third or fourth generation of those who hate him. This should not be taken, as some Jews in Ezekiel's day took it, that God punishes children for their parents' behavior, since that would violate God's own principle of justice (Ezek 18:2-3, Deut 24:16, 2 Kings 14:6; see also Ex 20:5-6). Ezekiel corrected this error by explaining that each person will be rewarded or judged for their own behaviors (Ezek 18:5-23). That said, children often do suffer as a consequence of their parents' sins. 'Third and fourth generation' could be shorthand for a household that consists of up to four generations: children, parents, grandparents and sometimes great-grandparents. The sin of any one of them negatively affects the whole household. For example, a mother's substance abuse might result in a child's birth defects, or a parent who gambles in excess may have no money to care for the family. Children may mimic the sinful behaviors of their parents. It is only insofar as the child continues in the sins of the parent that God warns he will punish successive generations for those sins." Joe M. Sprinkle, unpublished communication; see his teaching videos "The Ten Commandments," June 24, 2024, YouTube, 6:13, www.youtube.com/watch?v=EywekiX3V5M; and "Ezekiel Part 1," October 8, 2024, YouTube, 26:14, www.youtube.com/watch?v=lCc FFK00PoM.

[6]See Joni and Friends, www.joniandfriends.org.

[7]Letter written by C. S. Lewis to Sheldon Vanauken, in Sheldon Vanauken, *A Severe Mercy* (San Francisco: Harper & Row, 1978), 241.

[8]The Bible gives us additional examples of God displaying his work through individual medical issues. Elizabeth and Zacharias had no children, but their infertility occurred in order that the work of God might be displayed in their life well after Elizabeth's menopause (Lk 1:6-7). Hezekiah, a king of Israel, experienced a transformation in his faith due to an illness, as described in Isaiah 38, that affected his subsequent rule of the nation of Israel.

[9]Six types of spiritual care interventions in nursing practice have been described: compassionate presence, active listening, witness, prayer, Scripture, and Christian community. See Judith A. Shelly, Arlene B. Miller, and Kimberly H. Fenstrermacher, *Called to Care*, 3rd ed. (Downers Grove, IL: InterVarsity Press, 2021), chap. 14.

[10]As quoted to me by Pastor Bob Mason.

[11]Hugh Leftcastle, "What Is the Definition of Spiritual Nihilism?," Quora, www.quora.com /What-is-the-definition-of-spiritual-nihilism.

[12]Peter S. Williams, *I Wish I Could Believe in Meaning: A Response to Nihilism* (Southampton, UK: Damaris, 2004).

[13]Os Guinness, *Signals of Transcendence: Listening to the Promptings of Life* (Downers Grove, IL: InterVarsity Press, 2023).

[14]"Webinar: Dr Walt Larimore—Using a Spiritual History to Uncover Religious Struggle," ICMDA, YouTube, 53:01, www.youtube.com/watch?v=NVrU8OC2gdc&list=PLny32oC mvmF8JSWo-VpwvDV18bNE4gVVg&index=91.

[15]Matlock, *Faith For the Curious*, chap. 3.

[16]Simona Dai, interviewed by Jessica Mendoza, "China Wants More Babies. Many Women Are Saying No," *The Journal* (podcast), January 5, 2024, www.wsj.com/podcasts/the -journal/china-wants-more-babies-many-women-are-saying-no/2FB1D60F-8D81-4783 -A85B-F66E2AEA9879.

CHAPTER 6: HEALING AND REPENTANCE

[1]"Repentance," in *Baker's Evangelical Dictionary of Biblical Theology*, ed. Walter A. Elwell (Grand Rapids, MI: Baker Books, 1996), www.biblestudytools.com/dictionary /repentance/; "Metanoia," in *The NAS New Testament Greek Lexicon*, 1999, www.bible studytools.com/lexicons/greek/nas/metanoia.html.

[2]The Bible portrays repentance as an instinctual human response to an encounter with God (Job 42; Is 6).

[3]"The God of Jesus and the prophets saves completely by grace. He cannot be manipulated by religious and moral performance—he can only be reached through repentance." Timothy J. Keller, *The Reason for God: Belief in an Age of Skepticism* (New York: Penguin Books, 2008), 74.

[4]For an example of repentance as preventative medicine, see John 3:1-10.

[5]For a concise summary of how Christianity transformed healthcare in the ancient world, see Paul J. Hudson, *Healthcare and the Mission of God* (Tulsa, OK: Genesis, 2024), chap. 8. For an academic assessment, see Rodney W. Stark, *The Rise of Christianity: A Sociologist Reconsiders History* (Princeton, NJ: Princeton University Press, 2020).

[6]The Greek words for "sickness" and "healing" used in James 5 have a wide semantic range, reflecting the Bible's holistic view of personhood and health, and may refer to bodily or spiritual afflictions or healing. The seemingly categorical assurance of healing offered in this passage (and Jer 15:19; 2 Chron 7:14) should be read as describing the usual state of affairs and applying broadly to health but not as a guarantee of bodily healing (2 Cor 12:7-10; Heb 9:27). This passage suggests that repentance and prayer are part of our initial approach to sickness, not the last modality we turn to. The modern, Western experience that prayer for healing is often ineffective may be due to our nonbiblical use of such prayer, which we tend to offer only after exhausting other treatments and without simultaneous practice of repentance.

[7]See 1 Peter 5:5-7, which describes the process of transferring our cares to God. First Peter 5:7 is often quoted in isolation, but humbling ourselves before God (1 Pet 5:5-6) precedes releasing our cares.

[8]For more about these diagnostic signs of a cold heart, listen to Serge, *Sonship Audio Lectures* (Greensboro, NC: New Growth Press, 2013), https://newgrowthpress.com/small -group-study-resources/topical-bible-study-books/sonship-audio-lectures-on-mp3/.

[9]Stephanie Hooker, Anjoli Punjabi, Kacey Justesen, Lucas Boyle, and Michelle D. Sherman, "Encouraging Health Behavior Change: Eight Evidence-Based Strategies," *Family Practice Management* 25, no. 2 (2018): 31-36.

[10]For instance, the series of minibooks published by New Growth Press, https:// newgrowthpress.com/minibooks/.

CHAPTER 7: THE FEAR OF DEATH

[1]Timothy J. Keller, "Growing My Faith in the Face of Death," *Atlantic*, March 7, 2021, www .theatlantic.com/ideas/archive/2021/03/tim-keller-growing-my-faith-face-death/618219/.

[2]See, e.g., the story of Elijah's earthly end as told in 2 Kings 2:1-15, or the death of Moses recounted in Deuteronomy 34; compare with Paul's reflections in Philippians 1:22-25.

[3]See, e.g., the events leading to Uriah's death (2 Sam 11), Absalom's death (2 Sam 18), and the deaths of those killed by a collapsing tower (Lk 13).

[4]Here are two perspectives on God's role in determining the length of our lives:

"There is probably a difference between what a Calvinist and an Arminian would say on this topic, just as they would interpret Romans 8:28-30 differently. . . . From our perspective what we choose to do can lengthen or shorten our lives, as is obvious in the case of someone who commits suicide. God generally does not predestine each of our actions. Within certain bounds we have choices. But God foreknows what free choices we will make and so has (as it were metaphorically) written the days of our lives in his book, from birth to death." Dr. Joe Sprinkle, personal communication.

"We do see hospice patients hold on for important life events or to accomplish a goal. They then relax and die with some peace in knowing that they were able to be on earth and be part of that. That said, many declare a goal to be there for a wedding, birth or graduation and then do not survive to that time. My conclusion is that there *seems* to be a volitional aspect to dying but only God knows our days and his will for our lives." Dr. Kevin Whitford, personal communication.

[5]For a defense of the biblical promise of physical resurrection, see Nicholas T. Wright, *Surprised by Hope: Rethinking Heaven, Resurrection, and the Mission of the Church* (San Francisco: HarperOne, 2008).

[6]See Matthew McCullough, *Remember Death* (Wheaton, IL: Crossway, 2018), chap. 1.

[7]Ariane Froidevaux, Yoav S. Bergman, and Dikla Segel-Karpas, "Subjective Nearness-to-Death and Retirement Anxiety Among Older Workers: A Three-Way Interaction with Work Group Identification," *Research on Aging* 44, nos. 9-10 (2022): 770-81, https:// pubmed.ncbi.nlm.nih.gov/35344459/.

[8]Ernest Becker, *The Denial of Death* (New York: Free Press, 1973).

[9]Brian L. Burke, Andy Martens, and Erik H. Faucher, "Two Decades of Terror Management Theory: A Meta-analysis of Mortality Salience Research," *Personality and Social Psychology Review* 14, no. 2 (2010): 155-95, http://doi.org/10.1177/1088868309352321.

[10]Xiaoyu Zhou, Yafeng Pan, Ruqian Zhang, Litian Bei, and Xianchun Li, "Mortality Threat Mitigates Interpersonal Competition: An EEG-Based Hyperscanning Study," *Social Cognitive and Affective Neuroscience* 16, no. 6 (2021): 621-31, https://academic.oup.com/scan /article/16/6/621/6182540?login=false.

[11]Burke, Martens, and Faucher, "Two Decades of Terror Management Theory"; Gilad Hirschberger, Tom Pyszczynski, Tsachi Ein-Dor, Tal Shani Sherman, Eihab Kadah, Pelin Kesebir, and Young Chin Park, "Fear of Death Amplifies Retributive Justice Motivations and Encourages Political Violence," *Peace and Conflict Journal of Peace Psychology* 22, no. 1 (2016): 67-74, http://doi.org/10.1037/pac0000129; Goda Gegieckaite and Evaldas Kazlauskas, "Fear of Death and Death Acceptance Among Bereaved Adults: Associations with Prolonged Grief," *Omega—Journal of Death and Dying* 84, no. 3 (2022): 884-98, http://doi.org/10.1177/0030222820921045.

[12]Joel D. Lieberman and Jamie Arndt, "Terror Management Theory and Jury Decision-Making," *The Jury Expert*, July 1, 2009, https://thejuryexpert.com/2009/07/terror -management-theory-and-jury-decision-making/.

[13]Zainab Zahran, Khaldoun M. Hamdan, Ayman M. Hamdan-Mansour, Rabia S. Allari, Abeer A. Alzayyat, and Abeer M. Shaheen, "Nursing Students' Attitudes Towards Death and Caring for Dying Patients," *NursingOpen* 9, no. 1 (2022): 614-23, https://pubmed .ncbi.nlm.nih.gov/34729934/; Wen-Pei Chang and Yen-Kuang Lin, "Influence of Basic Attributes and Attitudes of Nurses Toward Death on Nurse Turnover: A Prospective Study," *International Nursing Review* 70, no. 2 (2023): 476-84, http://doi.org/10.1111 /inr.12781; Qiaohong Guo and Ruishuang Zheng, "Assessing Oncology Nurses' Attitudes Towards Death and the Prevalence of Burnout: A Cross-Sectional Study," *European Journal of Oncology Nursing* 42 (2019): 69-75, http://doi.org/10.1016/j.ejon.2019.08.002.

[14]Komal Meher, Mamoona Mushtaq, and Shameem Fatima, "Death Anxiety and Well-Being in Doctors During COVID-19: The Explanatory and Boosting Roles of Sleep Quality and Work Locality," *Omega (Westport)* 89, no. 2 (2022): 667-82, https://pmc.ncbi .nlm.nih.gov/articles/PMC8958309/.

[15]Dilek Anuk, Nilüfer Alçalar, Esra Kaytan Sağlam, and Güler Bahadir, "Breaking Bad News to Cancer Patients and Their Families: Attitudes Toward Death Among Turkish Physicians and Their Communication Styles," *Journal of Psychosocial Oncology* 40, no. 1 (2022): 115-30, http://doi.org/10.1080/07347332.2021.1969488.

[16]Michael Balboni, "Faith and Biomedicine in Dialogue," Veritas Forum, April 18, 2013, YouTube, 1:18:39, www.youtube.com/watch?v=Fh73NQfW-Ak.

[17]Meryem B. Bulut, "Relationship Between COVID-19 Anxiety and Fear of Death: The Mediating Role of Intolerance of Uncertainty Among a Turkish Sample," *Current*

Psychology 42, no. 10 (2023): 8441-50, https://pmc.ncbi.nlm.nih.gov/articles/PMC9159776/; Stephen Waite, Philip Hyland, Kate M. Bennett, Richard P. Bentall, and Mark Shevlin, "Testing Alternative Models and Predictive Utility of the Death Anxiety Inventory-Revised: A COVID-19 Related Longitudinal Population Based Study," *Acta Psychologica (Amsterdam)* 225 (May 2022): 103539, http://doi.org/10.1016/j.actpsy.2022.103539; Rachel E. Menzies, Louise Sharpe, and Ilan Dar-Nimrod, "The Relationship Between Death Anxiety and Severity of Mental Illnesses," *British Journal of Clinical Psychology* 58, no. 4 (2019): 452-67, http://doi.org/10.1111/bjc.12229.

[18]Ya-Ling Huang, Patsy Yates, Fred Arne Thorberg, and Chiung-Jung Wu, "Influence of Social Interactions, Professional Supports and Fear of Death on Adults' Preferences for Life-Sustaining Treatments and Palliative Care," *International Journal of Nursing Practice* 28, no. 4 (2022): e12940, http://doi.org/10.1111/ijn.12940.

[19]Selçuk Görücü and Gülşah Gürol Arslan, "The Investigation of Death Anxiety and Spiritual Well-Being Levels of Family Members of Patients Admitted to Intensive Care Unit," *Journal of Caring Sciences* 13, no. 1 (2024): 20-26, http://doi.org/10.34172/jcs.2024.33069.

[20]Jonathan Jong, "Death Anxiety and Religion," *Current Opinion in Psychology* 40 (August 2021): 40-44, http://doi.org/10.1016/j.copsyc.2020.08.004; Mahdi Rezapour, "The Interactive Factors Contributing to the Fear of Death," *Frontiers in Psychology* 13 (June 2022): 905594, http://doi.org/10.3389/fpsyg.2022.905594; Jonathan Jong, Robert Ross, Tristan Philip, Si-Hua Chang, Naomi Simons, and Jamin Halberstadt, "The Religious Correlates of Death Anxiety: A Systemic Review and Meta-analysis," *Religion, Brain & Behavior* 8, no. 1 (2018): 4-20, http://doi.org/10.1080/2153599X.2016.1238844.

[21]Nienke P. M. Fortuin, Johannes B. A. M. Schilderman, and Eric Venbrux, "Religion and Fear of Death Among Older Dutch Adults," *Journal of Religion, Spirituality & Aging* 31, no. 3 (2019): 236-54, http://doi.org/10.1080/15528030.2018.1446068; Hélio José Coelho-Júnior, Riccardo Calvani, Francesco Panza, Riccardo F. Allegri, Anna Picca, Emanuele Marzetti, and Vicente Paulo Alves, "Religiosity/Spirituality and Mental Health in Older Adults: A Systemic Review and Meta-analysis of Observational Studies," *Frontiers in Medicine (Lausanne)* 12, no. 9 (2022): 877213, http://doi.org/10.3389/fmed.2022.877213.

[22]Timothy J. Keller, *On Death* (New York: Penguin Books, 2020), chap. 1.

[23]McCullough, *Remember Death*, chap. 2.

[24]"Somehow" here refers not to the eventuality of resurrection but the means by which resurrection occurs.

[25]Subconscious fears may also be part of psychological and psychiatric illness and may merit expert professional care. This chapter speaks to the ubiquitous human fear of death and is not addressing particular psychological or psychiatric disorders such as thanatophobia.

[26]Atul Gawande, *Being Mortal* (New York: Holt, 2014).

[27]Tim Mackie and Jon Collins, "Jesus as the Ultimate Gift," *BibleProject* (podcast), August 26, 2019, https://bibleproject.com/podcast/jesus-ultimate-gift/.

CHAPTER 8: INTEGRITY

[1]The distinction between compassion and empathy, and the evidence linking compassion, quality of care, and career satisfaction, is discussed in more detail in chapter twelve.

[2]Chelsia Harris and Mary T. Quinn Griffin, "Nursing on Empty," *Journal of Christian Nursing* 32, no. 2 (2015): 80-87, http://doi.org/10.1097/CNJ.0000000000000155; Constance Guille and Srijan Sen, "Burnout, Depression, and Diminished Well-Being Among Physicians," *New England Journal of Medicine* 391 (2024): 1519-27, http://doi.org/10.1056/NEJMra2302878.

[3]Anna Garnett, Lucy Hui, Christina Oleynikov, and Sheila Boamah, "Compassion Fatigue in Healthcare Providers: A Scoping Review," *BMC Health Services Research* 23 (2023): 1336, https://pubmed.ncbi.nlm.nih.gov/37258070/.

[4]Kathleen Flarity, Ian Stanley, and Michael D. April, "Strengthening the Psychological Health and Readiness of Military Critical Care Nurses for Disaster and Future Combat Environments," *Critical Care Nursing* 44, no. 4 (2024): 53-57, http://doi.org/10.4037/ccn2024168; Jeffrey W. Katzman et al., "Caring for the Caregivers: Improving Mental Health Among Health Professionals Using the Behavioral Health Professional Workforce Resilience ECHO Program," *Healthcare (Basel)* 12, no. 17 (2024): 1741, http://doi.org/10.3390/healthcare12171741; Ana A. Chatham, Liana J. Petruzzi, Snehal Patel, W. Michael Brode, Rebecca Cook, Brenda Garza, Ricardo Garay, Tim Mercer, and Carmen R. Valdez, "Structural Factors Contributing to Compassion Fatigue, Burnout, and Secondary Traumatic Stress Among Hospital-Based Healthcare Professionals During the COVID-19 Pandemic," *Qualitative Health Research* 34, no. 4 (2023): 362-73, http://doi.org/10.1177/10497323231213825; Beth L. Muehlhausen, "Spirituality and Vicarious Trauma Among Trauma Clinicians: A Qualitative Study," *Journal of Trauma Nursing* 28, no. 6 (2021): 367-77, http://doi.org/10.1097/JTN.0000000000000616; Mackenzie N. Naert, Cassandra Pruitt, Alex Sarosi, Jill Berkin, Joanne Stone, and Andrea S. Weintraub, "A Cross-Sectional Analysis of Compassion Fatigue, Burnout, and Compassion Satisfaction in Maternal-Fetal Medicine Physicians in the United States," *American Journal of Obstetrics and Gynecology: Maternal-Fetal Medicine* 5, no. 7 (2023): 100989, http://doi.org/10.1016/j.ajogmf.2023.100989.

[5]Barry G. Webb, *Job*, Evangelical Biblical Commentary (Bellingham, WA: Lexham Academic, 2023).

[6]*Satan* is capitalized in the NIV, suggesting an individual spirit's name. The Hebrew word translated "Satan" in the first chapters of Job may also mean "adversary" or "prosecutor," and there is scholarly disagreement about the meaning of *Satan* in the context of Job. See Michael S. Heiser, *The Unseen Realm: Recovering the Supernatural Worldview of the Bible* (Bellingham, WA: Lexham, 2015), chap. 27.

[7]Wissem Hafsi and Siva Naga S. Yarrarapu, "Job Syndrome," in *StatPearls [Internet]*, August 28, 2023, www.ncbi.nlm.nih.gov/books/NBK525947/.

[8]The Hebrew word *hesed*, which can be translated as "faithfulness," "favor," or "unchanging love," is often used in reference to God. He displays steadfast love toward all of his creation (Ps 145:14-16; Jn 3:16).

[9]The Bible does give us glimpses into God's purposes in human suffering—glimpses that demonstrate that suffering can have beneficial outcomes. Broadly speaking, God may use suffering for good in the life of the suffering person or in the lives of others. See Genesis 50:20; Jeremiah 17:7-8; Matthew 6:30; 13:1-23; John 15:1-2; Romans 5:3-5; 8:28; 2 Corinthians 4:7-12; Galatians 4:13-14; 5:22-23; Philippians 3:10-11; Hebrews 12:7-11; 13:15.

[10]See Job 1:6-12; 2:1-6, where God gives Job over into Satan's hands.

[11]Jeannie L. Gribben, Samuel M. Kase, Elisha D. Waldman, and Andrea S. Weintraub, "Cross-Sectional Analysis of Compassion Fatigue, Burnout and Compassion Satisfaction in Pediatric Critical Care Physicians in the United States," *Pediatric Critical Care Medicine* 20, no. 3 (2019): 213-22, http://doi.org/10.1097/PCC.0000000000001803.

[12]Nicholas T. Wright, "Mind, Spirit, Soul and Body: All for One and One for All; Reflections on Paul's Anthropology in His Complex Contexts" (lecture, Society of Christian Philosophers, Fordham University, March 18, 2011), https://ntwrightpage.com/2016/07/12/mind-spirit-soul-and-body.

[13]Timothy J. Keller, "Worship," sermon preached at Redeemer Presbyterian Church, New York, New York, July 2, 2002, https://www.youtube.com/watch?v=PswZTmSIpv4.

[14]The ProQoL is available at https://proqol.org/proqol-measure.

CHAPTER 9: LAMENT

[1]William Ardill, *Journey On a Dusty Road* (N.p.: CreateSpace, 2016), 319-29.

[2]Michael Brennan Dick, "The Legal Metaphor in Job 31," *Catholic Biblical Quarterly* 41, no. 1 (1979): 37-50; Bruce Wells and F. Rachel Magdalene, "Law," in *Dictionary of the Old Testament: Wisdom, Poetry and Writings*, ed. Tremper Longman and Peter Enns (Downers Grove, IL: InterVarsity Press, 2008), 422-23.

[3]Mark Talbot, *When the Stars Disappear*, vol. 1, *Help and Hope from Stories of Suffering in Scripture* (Wheaton, IL: Crossway, 2020), 31. Scholars vary in their interpretation of the middle section of Job. Talbot's insights, as I understand them, are the basis for the view presented here.

[4]Numerous authors have analyzed the lament form. The elements of lament listed here are abstracted from Mark Talbot, *When the Stars Disappear*; Cameron Cole, "How to Prepare for Tragedy," *TGC Podcast*, August 28, 2020, www.thegospelcoalition.org/podcasts/tgc-podcast/how-to-prepare-for-tragedy/; Mark Vroegop, "How to Lament Well," Desiring God, accessed December 28, 2024, www.desiringgod.org/articles/dare-to-hope-in-god.

[5]Timothy J. Keller, "Praying the Gospel," (Sermon preached at Redeemer Presbyterian Church, New York, New York, March 19, 2000).

[6]Timothy J. Keller, "Suffering: If God Is Good, Why Is There So Much Evil in the World?" (sermon preached at Redeemer Presbyterian Church, New York, October 1, 2006),

https://gospelinlife.com/sermon/suffering-if-god-is-good-why-is-there-so-much-evil-in
-the-world/.

[7]Mark Vroegop, "Lament Leads to Praise," accessed December 28, 2024, www.markvroe
gop.com/blog/lament-leads-to-praise.

[8]Ardill, *Journey on a Dusty Road*, 319.

[9]Talbot, *When the Stars Disappear*, 46-55.

[10]Talbot, *When the Stars Disappear*, 53.

[11]Ardill, *Journey on a Dusty Road*, 394.

CHAPTER 10: WHEN WE ASK, "WHY?" GOD SAYS, "WHO!"

[1]Ethan Helm, "Fighting Demons, Fighting Cancer" (undergraduate thesis), 2007, Lake Forest College.

[2]Does scientific progress invalidate this part of God's argument? Since Job's time, people have discovered many of the laws and mechanisms through which God created and sustains our world. Science is a kingly endeavor (Prov 25:2), but we do not share in God's role as creator and sustainer of creation (Heb 1:1-3). The extent of his knowledge of us, our world, and the arc of our lives remains qualitatively different from our knowledge and understanding. He designed and made the organs we know and the bodies treat (Ps 139:13). No matter how thorough our knowledge becomes or how kingly our scientific insights are, we did not create the biological laws and components that are the basis for life, and therefore we do not have standing to question God's purposes and plans in creation.

[3]Timothy J. Keller, "Relying on the Law" (sermon preached at Redeemer Presbyterian Church, New York, December 14, 1997), https://podcast.gospelinlife.com/e/relying -on-the-law/.

[4]Mark Talbot, personal communication.

[5]Talbot, personal communication.

[6]Jesus' sacrifice for us affords us access to God (Mt 27:52; Heb 6:19; 10:20).

[7]Mark Talbot, *Give Me Understanding That I May Live: Situating Our Suffering Within God's Redemptive Plan* (Wheaton, IL: Crossway, 2022).

[8]Helm, "Fighting Demons, Fighting Cancer."

CHAPTER 11: HEALING AND THE GOSPEL

[1]N. T. Wright writes of his similar experience with regard to the gospel as it is presented in the Gospels: "I had stumbled, without realizing it, on a weak spot in the general structure of Christian faith as it has come to be expressed in today's world." Wright, *How God Became King: The Forgotten Story of the Gospels* (San Francisco: HarperOne, 2016), 5. I've benefited from his analysis.

[2]Mark Matlock, *Faith for the Curious: How an Era of Spiritual Openness Shapes the Way We Live and Helps Others Follow Jesus* (Grand Rapids, MI: Baker Books, 2024), chap. 7.

[3]I'm indebted to Dr. Rachel Nunn and the Saline Process curriculum for linking these three biblical images.

[4]David A. Fryburg, Steven D. Ureles, Jessica G. Myrick, Francesca Dillman Carpentier, and Mary Beth Oliver, "Kindness Media Rapidly Inspires Viewers and Increases Happiness, Calm, Gratitude, and Generosity in a Healthcare Setting," *Frontiers in Psychology* 11 (2021), 591942, https://www.frontiersin.org/journals/psychology/articles/10.3389/fpsyg.2020.591942/full.

[5]Adapted from "What We Value," Autumn Ridge Church, Rochester, MN, https://autumn ridge.church/about-us/.

CHAPTER 12: WHY JESUS WENT INTO HEALTHCARE

[1]"U.S. Physicians Overwhelmingly Satisfied with Career Choice," American Medical Association, March 30, 2017, www.ama-assn.org/press-center/press-releases/survey-us -physicians-overwhelmingly-satisfied-career-choice; Lesley Wilkes, Leanne Corwin, and Maree Johnson, "The Reasons Students Choose to Undertake a Nursing Degree," *Collegian* 22, no. 3 (2015): 259-65, https://doi.org/10.1016/j.colegn.2014.01.003.

[2]Muthuraman Narayanasamy, Anand Ruban, and Prakash Somi Sankaran, "Factors Influencing to Study Medicine: A Survey of First-Year Medical Students from India," *Korean Journal of Medical Education* 31, no. 1 (2019): 61-71, https://pubmed.ncbi.nlm.nih .gov/30852862/.

[3]Sarita Silveira, Malvika Godara, and Tania Singer, "Boosting Empathy and Compassion Through Mindfulness-Based and Socioemotional Dyadic Practice: Randomized Controlled Trial with App-Delivered Trainings," *Journal of Medical Internet Research* 26, no. 25 (2023): e45027, http://doi.org/10.2196/45027.

[4]"Agape," in *The NAS New Testament Greek Lexicon*, 1999, www.biblestudytools.com /lexicons/greek/nas/agape.html.

[5]Katherine J. Holzer, Harshavardhan Bollepalli, Jennifer Carron, Lauren H. Yaeger, Michael S. Avidan, Eric J. Lenze, and Joanna Abraham, "The Impact of Compassion-Based Interventions on Perioperative Anxiety and Depression: A Systematic Review and Meta-analysis," *Journal of Affective Disorders* 365 (November 2024): 476-91, http://doi .org/10.1016/j.jad.2024.08.110; Claudia Ferrreira et al., "Randomized Controlled Trial of an Acceptance and Commitment Therapy and Compassion-Based Group Intervention for Persons with Inflammatory Bowel Disease: The LIFEwithIBD Intervention," *Frontiers in Psychology* 15 (2024): 1367913, http://doi.org/10.3389/fpsyg.2024.1367913; KariAnne R. Vrabel, Glenn Waller, Ken Goss, Bruce Wampold, Maren Kopland, and Asle Hoffart, "Cognitive Behavioral Therapy Versus Compassion Focused Therapy for Adult Patients with Eating Disorders with and Without Childhood Trauma: A Randomized Controlled Trial in an Intensive Treatment Setting," *Behavioral Research and Therapy* 174 (March 2024): 104480, http://doi.org/10.1016/j.brat.2024.104480.

[6]"Report of the Mid Staffordshire NHS Foundation Trust Public Inquiry," UK Stationery Office, February 6, 2013, www.gov.uk/government/publications/report-of-the-mid -staffordshire-nhs-foundation-trust-public-inquiry.

[7]NHS Commissioning Board, "Compassion in Care," December 2012, www.england.nhs
.uk/wp-content/uploads/2012/12/compassion-in-practice.pdf.

[8]Jane Cummings, "Compassion in Practice: Evidencing the Impact," National Health
Service, May 2016, www.england.nhs.uk/wp-content/uploads/2016/05/cip-yr-3.pdf.

[9]Netta Weinstein and Richard Ryan, "When Helping Helps: Autonomous Motivation for
Prosocial Behavior and Its Influence on Well-Being for the Helper and Recipient,"
Journal of Personality and Social Psychology 98, no. 2 (2010): 222-44, https://pubmed
.ncbi.nlm.nih.gov/20085397/.

[10]Natália Ondrejková and Júlia Halamová, "Prevalence of Compassion Fatigue Among
Helping Professions and Relationship to Compassion for Others, Self-Compassion and
Self-Criticism," *Health and Social Care in the Community* 30 (2022): 1680-94, https://
pubmed.ncbi.nlm.nih.gov/35133041/; Sajad Khanjani, Yousef Asmari Bardezard,
Aliakbar Foroughi, and Fayegh Yousefi, "Burnout, Compassion for Others and Fear of
Compassion: A Quantitative Study in Iranian Nurses," *Trends in Psychiatry and Psycho-
therapy* 43, no. 3 (2021): 193-99, https://pubmed.ncbi.nlm.nih.gov/34882362/.

[11]Constance Guille and Srijan Sen, "Burnout, Depression, and Diminished Well-Being
Among Physicians," *New England Journal of Medicine* 391 (2024): 1519-27, https://www
.nejm.org/doi/full/10.1056/NEJMra2302878.

[12]Yasser Rezapour-Mirsaleh, Fatemah Abolhasani, Raziyeh Amini, Mohammed Javad
Rezai, Azadeh Choobforoushzadeh, and Leila Shameli, "Effects of Religious Versus Non-
religious Self-Compassion Interventions on Anxiety and Quality of Life of Iranian In-
fertile Women: A Randomized Controlled Trial," *Journal of Religion and Health*
(April 2024), https://pubmed.ncbi.nlm.nih.gov/38625638/.

[13]The Holy Spirit is here referred to using the Greek word *paraklētos*, meaning "one who
comes alongside to help."

[14]Susan Johnson, *Hold Me Tight* (Boston: Little Brown Spark, 2008).

CHAPTER 13: HOW MUCH FAITH IS ENOUGH?

[1]Sigurlaug H. Hafliðadóttir, Carsten B. Juhl, Sabrina M. Nielsen, Marius Henriksen, Ian
A. Harris, Henning Bliddal, and Robin Christensen, "Placebo Response and Effect in
Randomized Clinical Trials: Meta-research with Focus on Contextual Effects," *Trials* 22
(2021): 493, https://pubmed.ncbi.nlm.nih.gov/34311793/.

[2]In Luke's version of this account, Jesus both casts out a demon and heals the boy (Lk 9:42).
R. C. Sproul suggests that the boy had both epilepsy and demon possession: "When Satan
does come into a person's life, he uses whatever frailty is there to exploit his power over
his victim." "The Healing of the Possessed Boy" (sermon), https://www.youtube.com
/watch?v=CJK_7AttGEc.

[3]Timothy J. Keller, "Faith and Proof" (lecture, New York, March 7, 2019), https://podcasts
.apple.com/us/podcast/questioning-christianity-with-tim-keller/id1619691030?i=1000
559451444.

4Mark Matlock, *Faith for the Curious: How an Era of Spiritual Openness Shapes the Way We Live and Helps Others Follow Jesus* (Grand Rapids, MI: Baker Books, 2024), chap. 4.

5Matlock, *Faith for the Curious*, chap. 6.

6Leanne Roberts, Irshad Ahmed, Steve Hall, and Andrew Davison, "Intercessory Prayer for the Alleviation of Ill Health," *Cochrane Database of Systematic Reviews* 2009, CD000368, https://pmc.ncbi.nlm.nih.gov/articles/PMC7034220/.

7See, for instance, Eric C. Shattuck and Michael P. Muehlenbein, "Religiosity/Spirituality and Physiological Markers of Health," *Journal of Religion and Health* 59 (2020), 1035-54, doi: 10.1007/s10943-018-0663-6; Havva Sert, Merve Gulbahar Eren, Aylin Meşe Tunç, Kübra Üçgül, and Ayşe Çevirme, "Effectiveness of Spiritual and Religious Interventions in Patients with Cardiovascular Diseases: A Systematic Review of Meta-analysis of Randomized Controlled Trials," *Health Psychology* 44 (2024), 87-100, https://pubmed.ncbi.nlm.nih.gov/39325431/; Margarida Jarego et al., "Are Prayer-Based Interventions Effective Pain Management Options? A Systematic Review and Meta-analysis of Randomized Controlled Trials," *Journal of Religion and Health* 62 (2023), 1780-1809, https://pubmed.ncbi.nlm.nih.gov/35500682/.

8Al Weir, *Whispers in the Wind* (Bristol, TN: Christian Medical and Dental Associations, 2016), entry for January 24.

9Michael J. Balboni et al., "'It Depends': Viewpoints of Patients, Physicians, and Nurses on Patient-Practitioner Prayer in the Setting of Advanced Cancer," *Journal of Pain and Symptom Management* 41, no. 5 (2011): 836-47, https://pubmed.ncbi.nlm.nih.gov/21276700/.

Scripture Index